Glial Neurobiology

Glial Neurobiology

A Textbook

Alexei Verkhratsky
University of Manchester

Arthur Butt
University of Portsmouth

John Wiley & Sons, Ltd

Other Wiley Editorial Offices

John Wiley & Sons Inc., 111 River Street, Hoboken, NJ 07030, USA

Jossey-Bass, 989 Market Street, San Francisco, CA 94103-1741, USA

Wiley-VCH Verlag GmbH, Boschstr. 12, D-69469 Weinheim, Germany

John Wiley & Sons Australia Ltd, 33 Park Road, Milton, Queensland 4064, Australia

John Wiley & Sons (Asia) Pte Ltd, 2 Clementi Loop #02-01, Jin Xing Distripark, Singapore 129809

John Wiley & Sons Canada Ltd, 6045 Freemont Blvd, Mississauga, Ontario, L5R 4J3

Wiley also publishes its books in a variety of electronic formats. Some content that appears in print may
not be available in electronic books.

Anniversary Logo Design: Richard J. Pacifico

Library of Congress Cataloging in Publication Data

Verkhratskii, A. N. (Aleksei Nestorovich)
   Glial neurobiology : a textbook / Alexei Verkhratsky, Arthur Butt.
      p.   ;   cm.
   Includes bibliographical references and index.
   ISBN 978-0-470-01564-3 (cloth : alk. paper)
   1. Neuroglia.   I. Butt, Arthur.   II. Title.
   [DNLM: 1. Neuroglia. WL 102 V519g 2007]
   QP363.2.V47 2007
   611'.0188—dc22   2007015819

British Library Cataloguing in Publication Data

A catalogue record for this book is available from the British Library

ISBN 978-0-470-01564-3 (HB)
ISBN 978-0-470-51740-6 (PB)

Typeset in 10.5/12.5pt Times by Integra Software Services Pvt. Ltd, Pondicherry, India

Transferred to Digital Print 2008

Dedicated to our Families

Contents

Preface

Contemporary understanding of brain organization and function follows the neuronal doctrine, which places the nerve cell and neuronal synaptic contacts at the very centre of the nervous system. This doctrine considers glia as passive supportive cells, which are not involved in the informational exchange, and therefore secondary elements of the nervous system.

In the last few decades, however, our perception of the functional organization of the brain has been revolutionized. New data forces us to reconsider the main postulate of the neuronal doctrine – that neurones and synapses are the only substrate of integration in the central nervous system. We now learn that astroglial cells, which are the most numerous cells in the brain, literally control the naissance, development, functional activity and death of neuronal circuits. Astroglial cells are in fact the stem elements from which neurones are born. They also create the compartmentalization of the CNS and integrate neurones, synapses, and brain capillaries into inter-dependent functional units. Furthermore, astroglial cells form a functional syncytium, connected through gap junction bridges, which provides an elaborate intercellular communication route. This allows direct translocation of ions, metabolic factors and second messengers throughout the CNS, thereby providing a sophisticated means for information exchange. In a way the binary coded electrical communication within neuronal networks may be considered as highly specialized for rapid conveyance of information, whereas astroglial cells may represent the true substance for information processing, integration and storage. Will this truly heretical theory which subordinates neurones to glia be victorious at the end? Forthcoming years hold the answer.

When writing this book we have attempted to create a concise yet comprehensive account of glial cells and their role in physiology and pathology of the nervous system. We hope very much that this account may help the reader to discover a fascinating world of brain 'secondary' cells, which in fact are essential elements of the nervous system, whose functions and importance are yet to be fully appreciated.

Alexei Verkhratsky
Arthur Butt

List of abbreviations

AC	adenylate cyclase
ACh	acetylcholine
AIDS	acquired immunodeficiency syndrome
AMPA	α-amino-3-hydroxy-5-methyl-γ-isoxazolepropionate
AQP	aquaporins (water channels)
ATP	adenosine triphosphate
BDNF	brain-derived neurotrophic factor
BK	bradykinin
cAMP	cyclic adenosine monophosphate
cGMP	cyclic guanosine monophosphate
Ca_V	voltage-gated calcium channels
CNP	2,3-cyclic nucleotide-3-phosphodiesterase
CNS	central nervous system
COX	cyclooxygenase
CSF	cerebrospinal fluid
DAG	diacylglycerol
E_K, E_{Na}, E_{Ca}, E_{Cl}	equilibrium potential for K^+, Na^+, Ca^{2+} and Cl^- respectively
EAAT	excitatory amino acid transporter
EM	electron microscopy
ET	endothelin
GABA	γ-aminobutiric acid
GC	guanilate cyclase
GFAP	glial acidic fibrillary protein
HIV	human immunodeficiency virus
$InsP_3$	inositol (1,4,5) trisphosphate
$InsP_3R$	inositol (1,4,5) trisphosphate receptor
K_{ir}	inwardly rectifying K^+ channels

KA	kainate
NAADP	nicotinic acid adenine dinucleotide phosphate
Na_V	voltage-gated sodium channels
NCX	sodium–calcium exchanger
NGF	nerve growth factor
NMDA	N-methyl-D-aspartate
OPC	oligodendrocyte precursor cells
PAF	platelet-activating factor
PLC	phospholipase C
PLP	proteolipid protein
PMCA	plasmalemmal calcium ATPase
PNS	peripheral nervous system
RyR	ryanodine receptor
SERCA	sarco(endo)plasmic reticulum calcium ATPase
V_m	membrane potential
$[Ca^{2+}]_i$	intracellular free calcium concentration
$[K^+]_o, [Na^+]_o, [Ca^{2+}]_o, [Cl^-]_o$	extracellular concentrations of potassium, sodium, calcium and chloride respectively
$[K^+]_i, [Na^+]_i, [Ca^{2+}]_i, [Cl^-]_i$	intracellular concentrations of potassium, sodium, calcium and chloride respectively

PART I

Physiology of Glia

1

Introduction to Glia

There are two major classes of cells in the brain – *neurones* and *glia* (Figure 1.1). The fundamental difference between these lies in their electrical excitability – neurones are electrically excitable cells whereas glia represent nonexcitable neural cells. Neurones are able to respond to external stimulation by generation of a plasmalemmal 'all-or-none' action potential, capable of propagating through the neuronal network, although not all neurones generate action potentials. Glia are unable to generate an action potential in their plasma membrane (although they are able to express voltage-gated channels). Glial cells are populous (as they account for ~90 per cent of all cells in the human brain) and diverse. In the central nervous system (CNS) they are represented by three types of cells of neural (i.e. ectodermal) origin, often referred to as 'macroglial cells' (which may also be properly called 'neuroglial cells'). These are the *astrocytes*, the *oligodendrocytes* and the *ependymal* cells. The ependymal cells form the walls of the ventricles in the brain and the central canal in the spinal cord. Ependymal cells are involved in production and movement of cerebrospinal fluid (CSF), in forming a separating layer between the CSF and CNS cellular compartments, and in exchange of substances between the two compartments. In addition to neuroglia, the umbrella term glia covers *microglia*, which are of non-neuronal (mesodermal) origin and originate from macrophages that invade the brain during early development and settle throughout the CNS. In the peripheral nervous system (PNS), the main class of glia is represented by *Schwann cells*, which enwrap and myelinate peripheral axons; other types of peripheral glia are satellite cells of sensory and sympathetic ganglia and glial cells of the enteric nervous system (ENS) of the gastrointestinal tract.

1.1 Founders of glial research: from Gabriel Valentin to Karl-Ludwig Schleich

The idea of the co-existence of active (excitable) and passive (non-excitable) elements in the brain was first promulgated in 1836 by the Swiss professor of

Glial Neurobiology: A Textbook Alexei Verkhratsky and Arthur Butt
© 2007 John Wiley & Sons, Ltd ISBN 978-0-470-01564-3 (HB); 978-0-470-51740-6 (PB)

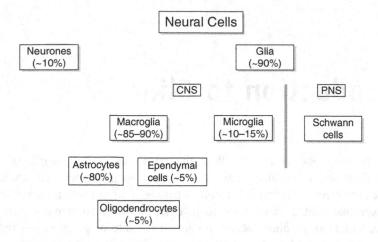

Figure 1.1 Neural cell types

anatomy and physiology Gabriel Gustav Valentin (1810–1883), in the book *Über den Verlauf und die letzten Enden der Nerven.* The concept and term 'glia' was coined in 1858 by Rudolf Ludwig Karl Virchow (1821–1902, Figure 1.2), in his own commentary to the earlier paper 'Über das granulierte Ansehen der Wandungen der Gehirnventrikel' (published in the journal *Allgemeine Zeitshrift fur Psychiatrie*; Vol. 3, pp. 242–250), and elaborated in detail in his book, *Die Cellularpathologie in ihrer Begründung auf physiologische und pathologische Gewebelehre.* Virchow was one of the most influential pathologists of the 19th century – he was one of the originators of the cellular theory (*'Omnis cellula e cellula'*) and of cellular pathology.

Virchow derived the term 'glia' from the Greek 'γλια' for something slimy and of sticky appearance (the root appeared in a form γλοιοσ in writings of Semonides where it referred to 'oily sediment' used for taking baths; in works of Herodotus, for whom it meant 'gum'; and in plays of Aristophanes, who used it in a sense of 'slippery or knavish'. In Modern Greek, the root remains in the word 'γλοιωης', which means filthy and morally debased person.) Virchow contemplated glia as a 'nerve putty' in 1858 when he held a chair of pathological anatomy at Berlin University. He initially defined glia as a 'connective substance, which forms in the brain, in the spinal cord, and in the higher sensory nerves a sort of *nervenkitt (neuroglia)*, in which the nervous system elements are embedded'; where 'nervenkitt' means 'neural putty'. For Virchow, glia was a true connective tissue, completely devoid of any cellular elements.

The first image of a neuroglial cell, the radial cell of the retina, was obtained by Heinrich Müller in 1851 – these are now known as retinal Müller cells. Several years later, these cells were also described in great detail by Max Schultze. In the beginning of 1860, Otto Deiters described stellate cells in white and grey matter, these cells closely resembling what we now know as astrocytes. Slightly

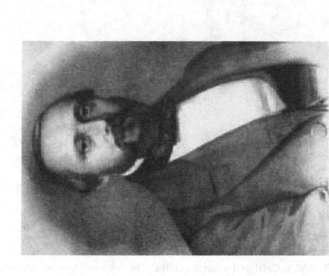

Rudolf VIRCHOW,
(1821–1902)

Figure 1.2 Rudolf Virchow – father of glia; the frontispiece of his book *Die Cellularpathologie in ihrer Begründung auf physiologische und pathologische Gewebelehre* (Berlin, Verlag von August Hirschfeld, 1858) is shown on the right

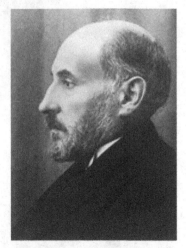

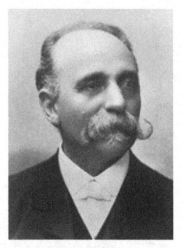

Santiago Ramón y Cajal   Camillo Golgi
(1852–1934)   (1843–1926)

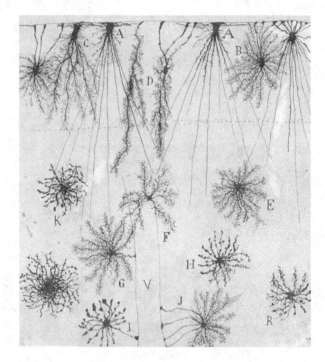

Figure 1.3 Santiago Ramón y Cajal and Camillo Golgi. The bottom panel shows original images of glial cells drawn by Ramón y Cajal: 'Neuroglia of the superficial layers of the cerebrum; child of two months. Method of Golgi. A, B, [C], D, neuroglial cells of the plexiform layer; E, F, [G, H, K], R, neuroglial cells of the second and third layers; V, blood vessel; I, J, neuroglial cells with vascular [pedicles].' This figure was reproduced as Figure 697 in *Textura* and Figure 380 in *Histologie*. (Copyright Herederos de Santiago Ramón y Cajal)

later (1869), Jakob Henle published the first image of cellular networks formed by stellate cells (i.e. astrocytes) in both grey and white matter of the spinal cord. Further discoveries in the field of the cellular origin of glial cells resulted from the efforts of many prominent histologists (Figures 1.3 and 1.4), in particular Camillo Golgi (1843–1926), Santiago Ramón y Cajal (1852–1934), and Pio Del Rio Hortega (1882–1945). S. Ramón y Cajal was born on May 1, 1852, in Aragon, Spain. In 1883 he was appointed Professor of Descriptive and General Anatomy at Valencia; in 1887 he was assumed a chair of in University of Barcelona and in 1892 he became Professor of Histology and Pathological Anatomy in Madrid.

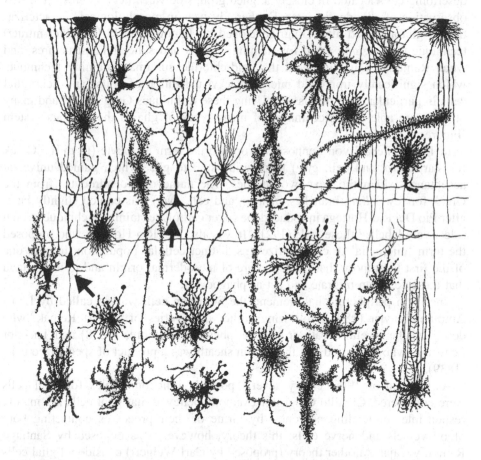

Figure 1.4 Morphological diversity and preponderance of glial cells in the brain as seen by Gustaf Magnus Retzius (1842–1919). Retzius was Professor of Histology at the Karolinska Institute in Stockholm from 1877. He investigated anatomy and histology of the brain, hearing organs and retina. The image shows a drawing from Retzius' book *Biologische Untersuchungen* (Stockholm: Samson and Wallin, 1890-1914), Vol. 6 (1894), Plate ii, Figure 5, where two neurones are marked with an arrow; the host of glial cells are stained by a silver impregnation method. (The image was kindly provided by Professor Helmut Kettenmann, MDC, Berlin)

Ramón y Cajal was, and remains, one of the most prominent and influential neurohistologists, who described fine structure of various parts of the nervous system. He was the most important supporter of the neuronal doctrine of brain structure. He won the Nobel Prize in 1906 together with Camillo Golgi.

Camillo Golgi was born in Brescia on July 7, 1843. Most of his life he spent in Pavia, first as a medical student, and then as Extraordinary Professor of Histology, and from 1881 he assumed a chair for General Pathology. He supported the reticular theory of brain organization. Using various ingenious staining and microscopic techniques, Camillo Golgi discovered a huge diversity of glial cells in the brain, and found the contacts formed between glial cells and blood vessels, as well as describing cells located in closely aligned groups between nerve fibres – the first observation of oligodendrocytes. Further advances in morphological characterization of glia appeared after Golgi developed his famous 'black' (or silver nitrate) technique (*la reazione nera*) for staining of cells and subcellular structures, and when Ramón y Cajal invented the gold-chloride sublimate staining technique, which significantly improved microscopic visualization of cells (and neuroglial cells in particular) in brain tissues. Using these techniques Golgi, Cajal and many others were able to depict images of many types of glia in the nervous system (Figures 1.3, 1.5).

In 1893, Michael von Lenhossek proposed the term astrocyte (from the Greek for star, *astro*, and cell, *cyte*) to describe stellate glia, which gained universal acceptance within the next two decades. The name oligodendrocyte (from the Greek for few, *oligo*, branches, *dendro*, and cell, *cyte*) was coined slightly later, after Pio Del Rio-Hortega introduced the silver carbonate staining technique, which selectively labelled these cells (1921). It was also Del Rio-Hortega who proposed the term 'microglia' to characterize this distinct cellular population; he was one of the first to propose that microglia are of mesodermal origin and to understand that these cells can migrate and act as phagocytes.

The main peripheral glial element, the Schwann cell, was so called by Louis Antoine Ranvier (1871), following earlier discoveries of Robert Remak, who described the myelin sheath around peripheral nerve fibres (1838) and Theodor Schwann, who suggested that the myelin sheath was a product of specialized cells (1839).

At the end of 19th century several possible functional roles for glial cells were considered. Camillo Golgi, for example, believed that glial cells are mainly responsible for feeding neurones, by virtue of their processes contacting both blood vessels and nerve cells; this theory, however, was opposed by Santiago Ramón y Cajal. Another theory (proposed by Carl Weigert) considered glial cells as mere structural elements of the brain, which filled the space not occupied by neurones. Finally, Santiago Ramón y Cajal's brother, Pedro, considered astrocytes as insulators, which prevented undesirable spread of neuronal impulses.

The idea of active neuronal–glial interactions as a substrate for brain function was first voiced in 1894 by Carl Ludwig Schleich (1859–1922) in his book *Schmerzlose Operationen* (Figure 1.5). Incidentally, this happened in the same

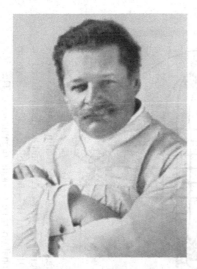

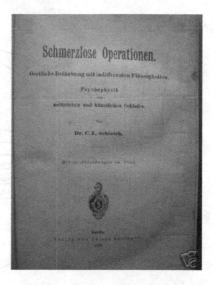

Carl Ludwig Schleich
(1859–1922)

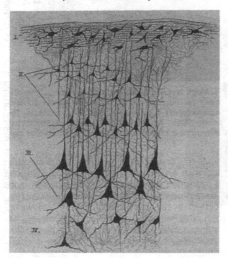

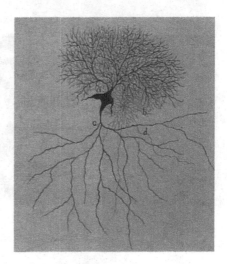

Figure 1.5 Carl Ludwig Schleich and the neuronal–glial hypothesis. Schleich was a pupil of Virchow and surgeon who introduced local anaesthesia into clinical practice. In 1894 he published a book *Schmerzlose Operationen. Betäubung mit indifferenten Flüssigkeiten*, Verlag Julius Springer, Berlin (the frontispiece of which is shown on the right upper panel). Apart from describing the principles of local anaesthesia, this also contained the first detailed essay on interactions in neuronal–glial networks as a substrate for brain function. Lower panels show original drawings from this book depicting intimate contacts between glial cells and neurones

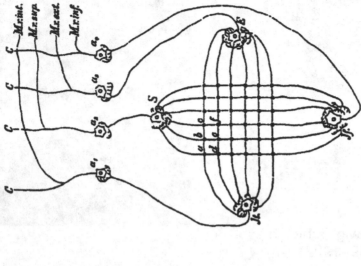

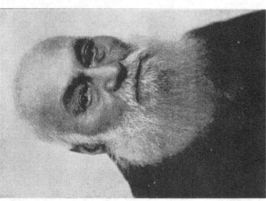

Wilhelm Gottfried
von Waldeyer
(1836–1921)

Sigmund Exner
(1846–1826)

Figure 1.6 The neuronal doctrine and its founders. Wilhelm Gottfried von Waldeyer was a professor of Anatomy in Berlin from 1883; where he made numerous important contributions to general histology (in particular he introduced the term 'chromosome'), and he also authored the term 'neurone' (1891). Sigmund Exner held a Chair in Physiology in Vienna University from 1891; and in 1894 he published a book (*Entwurf zur physiologischen Erklärung der psychishen Erscheinungen*, 1894), which described the neuronal doctrine of brain organization. The right panel displays an original scheme from his book, which shows neuronal networks connected by synapses

year as the 'neuronal' doctrine was promulgated by Sigmund Exner (1846–1926) in the book *Entwurf zur physiologischen Erklärung der psychishen Erschein-ungen*, (Berlin, 1894; Figure 1.6), and only three years after the term 'neurone' was coined by Wilhelm Gottfried von Waldeyer (1891, Figure 1.6). Schleich believed that glia and neurones were equal players and both acted as active cellular elements of the brain. He thought that glial cells represented the general inhibitory mechanism of the brain. According to Schleich, neuronal excitation is trans-mitted from neurone to neurone through intercellular gaps, and these interneuronal gaps are filled with glial cells, which are the anatomical substrate for control-ling network excitation/inhibition. He postulated that the constantly changing volume of glial cells represents the mechanism for control – swollen glial cells inhibit neuronal communication, and impulse propagation is facilitated when glia shrink.

1.2   Beginning of the modern era

The modern era in glial physiology began with two seminal discoveries made in the mid 1960s, when Steven Kuffler, John Nicolls and Richard Orkand (1966) demonstrated electrical coupling between glial cells, and Milton Brightman and Tom Reese (1969) identified structures connecting glial networks, which we know now as gap junctions. Nonetheless, for the following two decades, glial cells were still regarded as passive elements of the CNS, bearing mostly supportive and nutritional roles. The advent of modern physiological techniques, most notably those of the patch-clamp and fluorescent calcium dyes, has dramatically changed this image of glia as 'silent' brain cells.

1.3   Changing concepts: Glia express molecules of excitation

The first breakthrough discovery was made in 1984 when groups led by Helmut Kettenmann and Harold Kimelberg discovered glutamate and GABA receptors in cultured astrocytes and oligodendrocytes. Several years later, in 1990 Ann Cornell-Bell and Steve Finkbeiner found that astroglial cells are capable of long-distance communication by means of propagating calcium waves. These calcium waves can be initiated by stimulation of various neurotransmitter receptors in the astroglial plasma membrane.

Detailed analysis of the expression of these receptors performed during the last two decades demonstrated that glial cells, and especially astrocytes, are capable of expressing practically every type of neurotransmitter receptor known so far. Moreover, glial cells were found to possess a multitude of ion channels, which can be activated by various extracellular and intracellular stimuli. Thus, glial cells are endowed with proper tools to detect the activity of neighbouring neurones.

1.4   Glia and neurones in dialogue

Neurotransmitter receptors and ion channels expressed in glial cells turned out to be truly operational. It has now been shown in numerous experiments on various regions of the CNS and PNS that neuronal activity triggers membrane currents and/or cytosolic calcium signals in glial cells closely associated with neuronal synaptic contacts.

Finally, glial cells can also feed signals back to neurones, as they are able to secrete neurotransmitters, such as glutamate and ATP. This discovery resulted from the efforts of several research groups, and has led to the concept of much closer interactions between two circuits, neuronal and glial, which communicate via both chemical and electrical synapses.

2

General Overview of Signalling in the Nervous System

2.1 Intercellular signalling: Wiring and volume modes of transmission

The fundamental question in understanding brain function is: 'How do cells in the nervous system communicate?' At the very dawn of experimental neuroscience two fundamentally different concepts were developed. The 'reticular' theory of Camillo Golgi postulated that the internal continuity of the brain cellular network works as a single global entity, while the 'neuronal–synaptical' doctrine of Sigmund Exner, Santiago Ramón y Cajal and Charles Scott Sherrington implied that every neurone is a fully separate entity and cell-to-cell contacts are accomplished through a specialized structure (the synapse), which appears as the physical barrier (synaptic cleft) between communicating neurones (Figure 2.1). The latter theory postulated the focality of the intercellular signalling events, whereas Golgi thought about diffused transmission through the neural reticulum, which may affect larger areas of the CNS. The synaptic theory was victorious, yet the nature of the signal traversing the synaptic cleft was the subject of the second 'neuroscience' war, between followers of John Carew Eccles, who believed in purely electrical synapses, and supporters of Otto Loewi, Henry Dale and Bernhard Katz who championed chemical transmission. This clash of ideas lasted for about 20 years before Eccles yielded and fully accepted the chemical theory. For a while everything calmed down and the neuronal chemical synapse theory looked unassailable. The cornerstone of this theory implied focal information transfer through synapses, and the brain can be relatively simply modelled as a precisely wired system of logical elements. As usual, nature appeared more complicated than our theories, and now we have to admit that several different modes of cell-to-cell communication are operational within the CNS.

Glial Neurobiology: A Textbook   Alexei Verkhratsky and Arthur Butt
© 2007 John Wiley & Sons, Ltd   ISBN 978-0-470-01564-3 (HB); 978-0-470-51740-6 (PB)

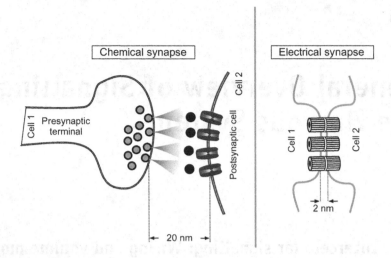

Figure 2.1 Chemical and electrical synapses. Signals between neural cells are transmitted through specialized contacts known as synapses (the word 'synapse' derives from term 'synaptein' introduced by C. Sherrington in 1897; this in turn was constructed from Greek 'syn-' meaning 'together' and 'haptein' meaning 'to bind').

In the case of chemical synapses, cells are electrically and physically isolated. The chemical synapse consists of presynaptic terminal, synaptic cleft ($\sim$20 nm in width) and postsynaptic membrane. The presynaptic terminal contains vesicles filled with neurotransmitter, which, upon elevation of intracellular free Ca^{2+} concentration within the terminal, undergo exocytosis and expel the neurotransmitter into the cleft. Neurotransmitter diffuses through the cleft and interacts with ionotropic and/or metabotropic receptors located on the postsynaptic membrane, which in turn results in activation of the postsynaptic cell.

In the case of electric synapses, adjacent cells are physically and electrically connected through trans-cellular gap junction channels, each formed by two connexons (see Chapter 5.4). The trans-cellular channels permit passage of ions, hence providing for the propagation of electrical signalling, as well as larger molecules, providing for metabolic coupling

Firstly, the direct physical connections between cells in the brain are of a ubiquitous nature. Gap junctions (Figure 2.1), which are in essence big intercellular channels, connect not only glial cells but also neurones, and possibly even neurones and glial cells. These gap junctions function as both electrical synapses (which allow electrotonic propagation of electrical signals) and as tunnels allowing intercellular exchange of important molecules such as second messengers and metabolites. Secondly, neurotransmitters released at synaptic terminals as well as extra-synaptically, and neuro-hormones secreted by a multitude of neural cells, act not only locally but also distantly, by diffusing through the extracellular space.

These discoveries led to an emergence of a new theory of cell-to-cell signalling in the nervous system, which combines highly localized signalling mechanisms (through chemical and electrical synapses), generally termed as a 'wiring transmission' (WT), with more diffuse and global signalling, which occur through diffusion in the extracellular space, as well as in the intracellular space within syncytial cellular networks; this way of signalling received the name of 'Volume Transmission' (VT), which can appear as extracellular (EVT) or intracellular (IVT). There are fundamental functional differences between wiring and volume transmission: wiring transmission is rapid (100s of microseconds to several seconds), is extremely local, always exhibits a one-to-one ratio (i.e. signals occurs only between two cells), and its effects are usually phasic (Figure 2.2). In contrast, volume transmission is slow (seconds to many minutes/hours), is global, exhibits a one-to-many ratio (i.e. substance released by one cell may affect a host of receivers), and its effects are tonic. Extracellular volume transmission in the CNS is rather well characterized, e.g. in open synapses, in signalling mediated by gaseous neurotransmitters such as nitric oxide (NO), in actions of neuropeptides, which are released extra-synaptically, in para-axonal transmission etc. (Figure 2.3). The concept of intracellular volume transmission is relatively new, and so far it is believed to be confined mostly to the astroglial syncytium. The substrate of intracellular volume transmission is represented by gap junctions. Gap junctions also form electrical synapses, which are a classical example of wiring transmission (very focal and extremely fast). Yet, the same channels are instrumental for long-distance

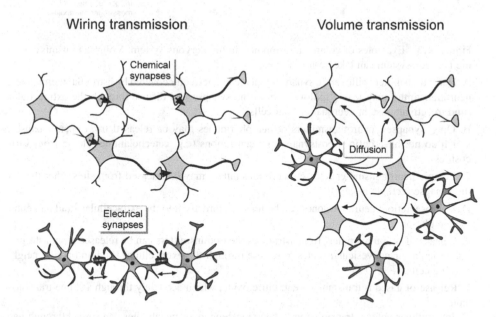

Figure 2.2 General principles of 'Wiring' and 'Volume' transmission. Wiring transmission is represented by chemical synapses, the most typical of the CNS; synapses are tightly ensheathed by astroglial membranes, which prevents spillover of neurotransmitter from the synaptic cleft, and ensures focal signal transfer (arrows). Wiring transmission is also accomplished by electrical synapses, which allow rapid and local transfer of electrical signals. Volume transmission is generally produced by the diffusion of neurotransmitter from a focal point to several cells

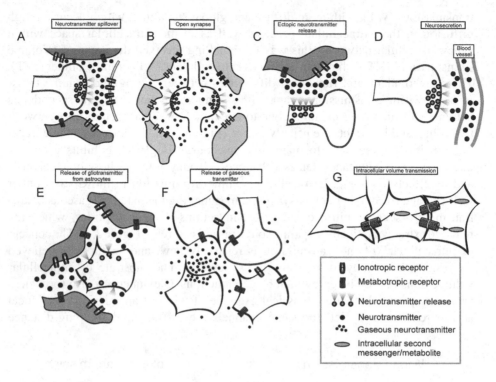

Figure 2.3 Examples of volume transmission in the nervous system. Volume transmission in the nervous system can take various routes:

A. Neurotransmitter spillover: in synapses that are not perfectly covered by astroglial membranes, neurotransmitter may leak ('spillover') from the synapse and diffuse through the extracellular fluid to activate distant neuronal or glial cells.

B. Open synapses: neurotransmitters or neurohormones may be released from open synapses, which do not have defined postsynaptic specializations (e.g. catecholamine release from varicosities).

C. Ectopic neurotransmitter release: neurotransmitters may be released from sites other than at the synapse (ectopic release).

D. Neurosecretion: neurohormones can be released directly into the extracellular fluid and enter the circulation.

E. Release of 'gliotransmitter' from astrocytes: neurotransmitters can be released from astroglia via vesicular or nonvesicular routes to diffuse through the extracellular fluid and act on neighbouring cells.

F. Release of gaseous transmitters: e.g. nitric oxide, which act solely through volume transmission.

G. Intracellular volume transmission: second messengers or metabolites can spread through gap junctions providing for intracellular volume transmission.

(Adapted and modified from Sykova E (2004) Extrasynaptic volume transmission and diffusion parameters of the extracellular space. *Neuroscience* **129**, 861–876; Zoli M, Jansson A, Sykova E, Agnati LF, Fuxe K (1999) Volume transmission in the CNS and its relevance for neuropsychopharmacology. *Trends Pharmacol Sci* **20**, 142–150) diffusion of molecules through glial networks, and as such they are involved in signal propagation on a one-to-many (cells) ratio. In fact, the same mechanism may be instrumental in neuronal networks, particularly in the developing CNS, as neuroblasts and immature neurones exhibit high levels of gap junctional coupling.

These three principal pathways of signal transmission in the brain, working in concert, underlie CNS information processing, by integration of all neural cells – neurones and glia – into highly effective information processing units. This is the concept of the functional neurone–glial unit.

2.2 Intracellular signalling

Intracellular signalling involves specific molecular cascades that sense, transmit and decode external stimuli. In the case of chemical neurotransmission, intracellular signalling invariably involves plasmalemmal *receptors* that sense the external stimulus, and effector systems, which can be located either within the plasmalemma

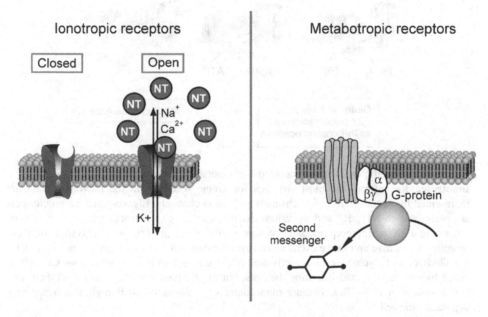

Figure 2.4 Ionotropic and metabotropic receptors. Ionotropic receptors are represented by ligand-gated ion channels. Neurotransmitter (NT) binding to the receptor site opens the channel pore, which results in ion fluxes; these in turn shift the membrane potential producing depolarization or hyperpolarization, depending on the ion and transmembrane electrochemical gradients. Metabotropic receptors belong to an extended family of seven-transmembrane-domain proteins coupled to numerous G-proteins. Activation of metabotropic receptors results in indirect opening of ion channels or in activation/inhibition of enzymes responsible for synthesis of different intracellular second messengers

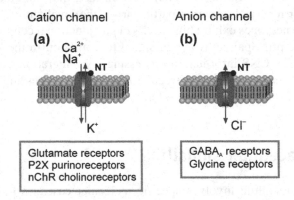

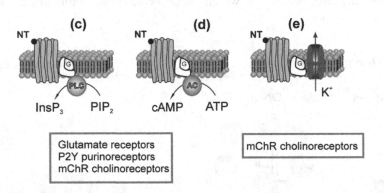

Figure 2.5 Specific examples of ionotropic and metabotropic receptors:
Ionotropic Receptors. The most abundant ionotropic receptors in the nervous system are represented by ligand-gated cation channels and anion channels. Ligand-gated cation channels are permeable to Na^+, K^+ and to various extents, Ca^{2+}, e.g. ionotropic glutamate receptors, ionotropic P2X purinoreceptors and nicotinic cholinoreceptors (nChRs); activation of these receptors depolarize and hence excite cells. Ligand-gated anion channels are permeable to Cl^-, e.g. $GABA_A$ and glycine receptors; activation of these receptors in neurones causes Cl^- influx, hence hyperpolarizing and inhibiting the cells, but in glia (and immature neurones) their activation results in Cl^- efflux, because intracellular Cl^- concentration is high, and hence they depolarize the cell.

Metabotropic Receptors. In the CNS, these are coupled to *phospholipase* C (PLC), *adenylate cyclase* (AC), and *ion channels*. Metabotropic receptors coupled to PLC produce the second messengers *InsP3* (inositol-1,4,5-trisphosphate) and *DAG* (diacylglycerol) from *PIP2* (phopshoinositide-diphosphate), e.g. group I metabotropic glutamate receptors and most P2Y metabotropic purinoreceptors. Metabotropic receptors coupled to AC produce *cAMP* (cyclic adenosine-monophosphate), e.g. group II and III metabotropic glutamate receptors, P2Y purinoreceptors, and some muscarinic cholinoreceptors (mChRs). Metabotropic receptors coupled to potassium channels are represented by muscarinic cholinoreceptors

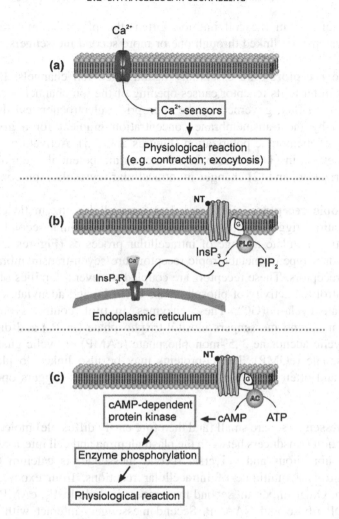

Figure 2.6 Examples of second messenger systems:

Calcium signalling system. Ca^{2+} ions enter the cytoplasm either through plasmalemmal Ca^{2+} channels or through intracellular Ca^{2+} channels located in the membrane of endoplasmic reticulum. Once in the cytoplasm, Ca^{2+} ions bind to numerous Ca^{2+}-sensitive enzymes (or Ca^{2+} sensors), to affect their activity and trigger physiological responses.

InsP3 signalling system. $InsP_3$, produced following activation of metabotropic receptors/PLC, binds to $InsP_3$ receptors (which are intracellular Ca^{2+} release channels) on the endoplasmic reticulum; activation of these receptors triggers Ca^{2+} release from intracellular stores and turns on the calcium signalling system.

cAMP signalling system. cAMP, produced following activation of metabotropic receptors/AC, binds to and activates a variety of cAMP-dependent protein kinases; these enzymes in turn phosphorylate effector proteins (e.g. plasmalemmal Ca^{2+} channels), thus affecting their function and regulating physiological cellular responses

(ion channels) or in the cell interior. Often, the plasmalemmal receptors and effector systems are linked through one or more second messengers.

Ionotropic receptors are essentially ligand-gated ion channels. Binding of a neurotransmitter to its receptor causes opening of the ion channel pore and generation of an ion flux, governed by the appropriate electrochemical driving force, determined by the transmembrane concentration gradient for a given ion and the degree of membrane polarization (Figures 2.4, 2.5). Activation of ionotropic receptors results in (1) a change in the membrane potential – depolarization or hyperpolarization, and (2) changes in intracellular (cytosolic) ion concentrations.

Metabotropic receptors are coupled to intracellular enzymatic cascades and their activation triggers the synthesis of various intracellular second messengers, which in turn regulate a range of intracellular processes (Figures 2.4, 2.5). The most abundant type of metabotropic receptors are seven-transmembrane-domain-spanning receptors. These receptors are coupled to several families of G-proteins, which control the activity of phospholipase C (PLC) and adenylate cyclase (AC) or guanylate cyclase (GC). These enzymes, in turn, control synthesis of the intracellular second messengers inositol-trisphosphate (InsP$_3$) and diacylglycerol (DAG), cyclic adenosine 3′,5′-monophosphate (cAMP) or cyclic guanosine 3′,5′-monophosphate (cGMP). The G-proteins may be also linked to plasmalemmal channels, and often activation of metabotropic receptors triggers opening of the latter.

Second messengers are small (and therefore easily diffusible) molecules that act as information transducers between the plasmalemma and cell interior (Figure 2.6). The most ubiquitous and universal second messenger is calcium (Ca^{2+} ions), which controls a multitude of intracellular reactions, from exocytosis to gene expression. Other important second messengers include InsP$_3$, cAMP and cGMP, cyclic ADP ribose and NAADP. Second messengers interact with intracellular receptors, usually represented by proteins/enzymes, and either up- or down-regulate their activity, therefore producing cellular physiological responses.

3

Morphology of Glial Cells

3.1 Astrocytes

Astrocytes (literally 'star-like cells') are the most numerous and diverse glial cells in the CNS. Some astrocytes indeed have a star-like appearance, with several primary (also called stem) processes originating from the soma, although astrocytes come in many different guises. An archetypal morphological feature of astrocytes is their expression of intermediate filaments, which form the cytoskeleton. The main types of astroglial intermediate filament proteins are *Glial Fibrillary Acidic Protein* (GFAP) and *vimentin*; expression of GFAP is commonly used as a specific marker for identification of astrocytes. The normal levels of GFAP expression, however, vary quite considerably: for example, GFAP is expressed by virtually every Bergmann glial cell in the cerebellum, whereas only about 15–20 per cent of astrocytes express GFAP in the cortex and hippocampus of mature animals.

Morphologically, the name astroglial cell is an umbrella term that covers several types of glial cell (Figures 3.1 and 3.2). The largest group are the 'true' astrocytes, which have the classical stellate morphology and comprise *protoplasmic astrocytes* and *fibrous astrocytes* of the grey and white matter, respectively. The second big group of astroglial cells are the *radial glia*, which are bipolar cells with an ovoid cell body and elongated processes. Radial glia usually produce two main processes, one of them forming endfeet on the ventricular wall and the other at the pial surface. Radial glia are a common feature of the developing brain, as they are the first cells to develop from neural progenitors; from very early embryonic stages radial glia also form a scaffold, which assist in neuronal migration. After maturation, radial glia disappear from many brain regions and transform into stellate astrocytes, although radial glia remain in the retina (*Müller glia*) and cerebellum (*Bergmann glia*). In addition to the two major groups of astroglial cells, there are smaller populations of specialized astroglia localized to specific regions of the CNS, namely the *velate astrocytes* of the cerebellum, the *interlaminar astrocytes* of the primate cortex, *tanycytes* (found in the periventricular organs, the hypophysis and the raphe part of the spinal cord), *pituicytes* in the neuro-hypophysis, and *perivascular* and *marginal astrocytes*. Finally, brain astroglia also

Glial Neurobiology: A Textbook   Alexei Verkhratsky and Arthur Butt
© 2007 John Wiley & Sons, Ltd   ISBN 978-0-470-01564-3 (HB); 978-0-470-51740-6 (PB)

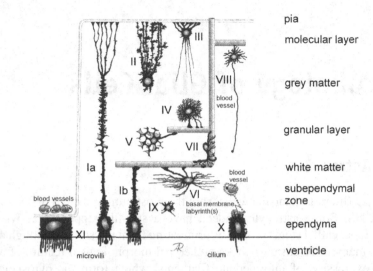

Figure 3.1 Morphological types of astrocytes; Ia – pial tanycyte; Ib – vascular tanycyte; II – radial astrocyte (Bergmann glial cell); III – marginal astrocyte; IV – protoplasmic astrocyte; V – velate astrocyte; VI – fibrous astrocyte; VII – perivascular astrocyte; VIII – interlaminar astrocyte; IX – immature astrocyte; X – ependymocyte; XI – choroid plexus cell. (From: Rechenbach A, Wolburg H (2005) Astrocytes and ependymal glia, In: *Neuroglia*, Kettenmann H & Ransom BR, Eds, OUP, p. 20.)

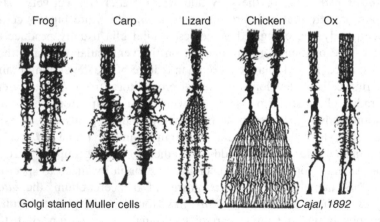

Figure 3.2 Müller cells from the retina of different species – Golgi stained cells as drawn by S. Ramón y Cajal

include several types of cells that line the ventricles or the subretinal space, namely *ependymocytes, choroid plexus cells* and *retinal pigment epithelial cells*.

1. *Protoplasmic astrocytes* are present in grey matter. They are endowed with many fine processes (on average ~50 µm long), which are extremely elaborated and complex. The processes of protoplasmic astrocytes contact blood vessels, forming so called 'perivascular' endfeet, and form multiple contacts with neurones. Some protoplasmic astrocytes also send processes to the pial surface, where they form 'subpial' endfeet. Protoplasmic astrocyte density in the cortex varies between 10 000 and 30 000 per mm^3; the surface area of their processes may reach up to 80 000 µm^2, and cover practically all neuronal membranes within their reach.

2. *Fibrous astrocytes* are present in white matter. Their processes are long (up to 300 µm), though much less elaborate compared to protoplasmic astroglia. The processes of fibrous astrocytes establish several perivascular or subpial endfeet. Fibrous astrocyte processes also send numerous extensions ('perinodal' processes) that contact axons at nodes of Ranvier, the sites of action potential propagation in myelinated axons. The density of fibrous astrocytes is ~200 000 cell per mm^3.

3. The retina contains specialized radial glia called *Müller cells*, which make extensive contacts with retinal neurones. The majority of Müller glial cells have a characteristic morphology (Figure 3.2), extending longitudinal processes along the line of rods and cones. In certain areas of retina, e.g. near the optic nerve entry site, Müller cells are very similar to protoplasmic astrocytes. In human retina, Müller glial cells occupy up to 20 per cent of the overall volume, and the density of these cells approaches 25 000 per mm^2 of retinal surface area. Each Müller cell forms contacts with a clearly defined group of neurones organized in a columnar fashion; a single Müller cell supports ~16 neurones in human retina, and up to 30 in rodents.

4. The cerebellum contains specialized radial glia called *Bergmann glia*. They have relatively small cell bodies (~15 µm in diameter) and 3–6 processes that extend from the Purkinje cell layer to the pia. Usually several (~8 in rodents) Bergmann glial cells surround a single Purkinje neurone and their processes form a 'tunnel' around the dendritic arborization of Purkinje neurones. The processes of Bergmann glial cells are extremely elaborated, and they form very close contacts with synapses formed by parallel fibres on Purkinje neurone dendrites; each Bergmann glial cell provides coverage for up to 8000 of such synapses.

5. *Velate astrocytes* are also found in the cerebellum, where they form a sheath surrounding granule neurones; each velate astrocyte enwraps a single granule neurone. A similar type of astrocyte is also present in the olfactory bulb.

6. *Interlaminar astrocytes* are specific for the cerebral cortex of higher primates. Their characteristic peculiarity is a very long single process (up to 1 mm) that extends from the soma located within the supragranular layer to cortical layer IV. The specific function of these cells is unknown, although they may be involved in delineating cortical modules spanning across layers.

7. *Tanycytes* are specialized astrocytes found in the periventricular organs, the hypophysis and the raphe part of the spinal cord. In the periventricular organs, tanycytes form a blood–brain barrier by forming tight junctions with capillaries (the blood–brain barrier is normally formed by tight junctions between the endothelial cells, but those in the periventricular organs are 'leaky', and the tanycytes form a permeability barrier between neural parenchyma and the CSF).

8. Astroglial cells in the neuro-hypophysis are known as *pituicytes*; the processes of these cells surround neuro-secretory axons and axonal endings under resting conditions, and retreat from neural processes when increased hormone output is required.

9. *Perivascular and marginal astrocytes* are localized very close to the pia, where they form numerous endfeet with blood vessels; as a rule they do not form contacts with neurones, and their main function is in forming the pial and perivascular *glia limitans barrier*, which assists in isolating the brain parenchyma from the vascular and subarachnoid compartments.

10. *Ependymocytes, choroid plexus cells* and *retinal pigment epithelial cells* line the ventricles or the subretinal space. These are secretory epithelial cells. They have been considered under the umbrella term glia because they are not neurones. The choroid plexus cells produce the CSF which fills the brain ventricles, spinal canal and the subarachnoid space; the ependymocytes and retinal pigment cells are endowed with numerous very small movable processes (microvilli and kinocilia) which by regular beating produce a stream of CSF and vitreous humour, respectively.

3.2 Oligodendrocytes

Oligodendroglia are glial cells with few processes, hence the prefix 'oligo'. The main function of oligodendrocytes (Figure 3.3) is the production of *myelin*, which insulates axons in the CNS, and assists fast saltatory action potential propagation (the same task is performed by Schwann cells in the PNS).

Oligodendrocytes were initially described by Del Rio Hortega in 1928; he classified these cells into four main phenotypes (I–IV) depending on their morphological appearance, and by the number of their processes and the size of the fibres they contacted. Del Rio Hortega also contemplated the main function of oligo-

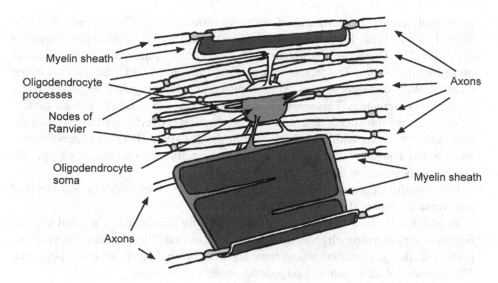

Figure 3.3 Oligodendrocyte and myelinated axons. Diagrammatic representation of a typical white matter oligodendrocyte based on intracellular dye-filled cells and electron microscopy. Each oligodendrocyte myelinates as many as 30–50 axons within 20–30 μm of the cell body. Along the axon, consecutive myelin sheaths separate nodes of Ranvier, the sites of action potential propagation. Each myelin sheath is a large sheet of membrane that is wrapped around the axon to form multiple lamellae and is connected to the cell body by fine processes

dendrocytes as producers of myelin for axonal insulation (this role was firmly proven only in 1964, after new electron microscopy techniques were introduced into neuro-histology).

Morphologically, type I and II oligodendrocytes are very similar; they have a small rounded cell body and produce four to six primary processes which branch and myelinate 10 to 30 thin (diameter <2 μm) axons, each secondary process forming a single internodal myelin segment of approximately 100–200 μm length, termed the internodal length (along axons, myelin sheaths are separated by nodes of Ranvier, which are small areas of unmyelinated axon where action potentials are generated; hence the distance between nodes is the *internode* and the length of a myelin segment between two nodes is the internodal length). Type I oligodendrocytes can be found in the forebrain, cerebellum, and spinal cord, whereas type II oligodendrocytes are observed only in white matter (e.g. corpus callossum, optic nerve, cerebellar white matter, etc.), where they are the primary cell type. Type III oligodendrocytes have a much larger cell body, and several thick primary processes, which myelinate up to five thick axons (4–15 μm in diameter), and produce myelin sheaths with approximately 200–500 μm internodal length; type III oligodendrocytes are located in the cerebral and cerebellar peduncles, the medulla oblongata and the spinal cord. Finally, type IV oligodendrocytes do not have processes, and form a single long myelin sheath (as great as 1000 μm internodal length) on the largest diameter axons; type IV oligodendrocytes are located almost exclusively around the entrances of the nerve roots into the CNS. During development, types I–IV are likely to originate from common oligodendrocyte progenitor cells (OPCs), which are multipolar cells that contact numerous small diameter premyelinated axons. The factors that regulate the fate of OPCs are unknown, but it seems likely that signals from axons of different calibre regulate oligodendrocyte phenotype divergence. This question is of some importance, because the dimensions of the myelin sheath determine the conduction properties of the axons in the unit, whereby axons with long thick myelin sheaths (type III/IV oligodendrocyte–axon units) conduct faster than those with short thin myelin sheaths (type I/II oligodendrocyte–axon units).

Oligodendrocytes also participate in the development of nodes of Ranvier and determine their periodicity (see Chapter 8).

In addition to these classical myelin-forming oligodendrocytes, a small population of nonmyelinating oligodendrocytes known as 'satellite oligodendrocytes' are present in the grey matter, where they are usually applied to neuronal perikaria. The function of these satellite oligodendrocytes is unknown.

3.3   NG2 expressing glia

In the 1980s, William Stallcup and colleagues identified a new population of cells in the adult CNS using antibodies to a novel chondroitin sulphate proteoglycan, NG2 (one of a series of molecules derived from mixed neurone (N) and glial (G) cultures). These NG2 immunopositive cells express many specific markers of oligodendrocyte progenitor cells (OPCs), e.g. platelet-derived growth factor alpha receptors (PDGFαR), and are generally considered to be oligodendroglial lineage cells. NG2 immunopositive cells do not co-express markers for mature oligodendrocytes (e.g. galactocerebroside, myelin-related proteins) or astrocytes (e.g. GFAP, vimentin, S100β, or glutamine synthetase). During development, NG2 immunopositive OPCs give rise to both myelinating oligodendrocytes and a substantial population (5–10 per cent of all glia) of NG2 positive cells that persist throughout the white and grey matter of the mature CNS. Hence, these cells are often called 'NG2-glia', and are characterized as having small somata and extending numerous thin, radially oriented processes, which branch two or more times close to their source. In the normal adult CNS, the vast majority (>90 per cent) of NG2-glia are not mitotically active, although they may become so in response to various insults. NG2-glia are able to generate oligodendrocytes during developmental remodelling of the CNS and following demyelination. NG2-glia may also generate neurones and astrocytes. Hence, NG2-glia may serve as multipotent adult neural stem cells. Nonetheless, the substantial majority of NG2-glia in the mature CNS appear to be fully differentiated, but like astrocytes (see below), appear to retain the function of stem cells in the brain throughout maturation and adulthood.

In the grey matter, NG2-glia form numerous contacts with surrounding neurones, and even receive neuronal afferents, which form functional synapses (see Chapter 6). In the white matter, NG2-glia are also characterized by complex morphology – they extend processes along myelinated axons, and often establish contacts with nodes of Ranvier, being in this respect similar to fibrous astrocytes. In addition to contacting neurones, NG2-glia form multiple associations with astrocytes and oligodendrocytes, and their myelin sheaths, as well as the subpial and perivascular *glia limitans*, but apparently NG2-glia do not form contacts with each other, and each cell has a 'territory' of about 200–300 μm in diameter. There is a clear morphological difference between NG2-glia in grey and white matter, whereby the former extend processes in all directions to form a symmetrical radial process arborization, whereas white matter NG2-glia have a polarized appearance and preferentially extend processes along axon bundles.

Physiologically, NG2-glia have several distinguishing properties – they express voltage-gated Na^+, Ca^{2+} and K^+ channels (yet they are generally unable to generate action potentials), as well as glutamate and GABA receptors, although not apparently glutamate transporters or glutamine synthetase, which distinguishes them from astrocytes. NG2-glia therefore are likely to actively communicate with neurones, with a particular task to monitor and rapidly respond to changes in neuronal activity. These cells were even named as '*synantocytes*' (from Greek συναντω *synanto*, meaning contact) to distinguish them from NG2 positive OPCs that generate oligodendrocytes during development, and to stress their distinct appearance, physiology and involvement in neuronal–glial interactions in the mature CNS. Notably, NG2-glia are highly reactive and rapidly respond to CNS insults by outgrowth and proliferation of processes. Activated NG2-glia participate in *glial scar* formation together with astrocytes. It has been postulated that a primary function of NG2-glia in the adult CNS may be to respond rapidly to changes in neural integrity, either to form a glial scar, or to generate neurones, astrocytes or oligodendrocytes, depending on the needs and the signals. NG2-glia are highly suited for these tasks via their multiple contacts with neural and glial elements.

3.4 Schwann cells

There are 4 types of Schwann cells in the PNS: *myelinating Schwann cells*, *nonmyelinating Schwann cells*, *perisynaptic Schwann cells* of the neuromuscular junction and *terminal Schwann-like cells* of the sensory neurites. All four types of Schwann cells originate from the neural crest (see Chapters 4 and 8) and during development they migrate along axons. Continuous contact with axons is particularly important as Schwann cell precursors die whenever such a contact is lost. With further developmental progress, the precursors turn into immature Schwann cells, which can survive without axons. These immature Schwann cells attach themselves to the nearest axons, which they start to ensheath. Schwann cells associated with a large diameter axon (≥1μm) begin to produce myelin and form an internodal myelin segment with a 1:1 ratio of Schwann cell:axon. Schwann cells attached to small diameter axons (<1 μm) do not form myelin, but produce a membrane sheath around a bundle of axons and separate the axons from each other within the nerve. The factors that regulate the fate of Schwann cells remain unknown, but (like oligodendrocytes) it is likely that these factors are produced by axons, and that axons of different calibre may produce distinct signals aimed at Schwann cells.

Myelinating Schwann cells also participate in forming nodes of Ranvier (see Chapter 8), and extend multiple perinodal processes that fill the nodal gap. Perinodal processes are internally connected through gap junctions formed by connexin 32 (Cx32). Perinodal processes form nodal gap substance and are involved in regulation of the ionic microenvironment around the node and, most likely, Schwann cell–axon interactions are important in Na^+ channels clustering at nodes and in stabilizing the structure of the nodal axonal membrane.

3.5 Microglia

Microglial cells are the immunocompetent cells residing in the CNS. In essence, microglia form the brain immune system, which is activated upon various kinds of brain injuries and diseases. Microglial cells represent about 10 per cent of all glial cells in the brain. Microglia are of a myelomonocytic origin, and the microglial precursor cells appear in the brain during early embryonic development. In the mature CNS, microglial cells may appear in three distinct states: the resting microglia, activated microglia and phagocytic microglia (see Chapter 9).

In the normal brain, microglial cells are present in the resting state, which is characterized by a small soma and numerous very thin and highly branched processes (hence these cells are also often called 'ramified'). The microglial cells reside in all parts of the brain, with the highest densities in the hippocampus, olfactory telencephalon, basal ganglia and substantia nigra. Every individual microglial cell is responsible for a clearly defined territory of about 50 000 μm^3 in volume; the processes of resting cells are never in contact with each other. There is a clear morphological difference between microglial cells residing in the grey versus white matter: the former extend processes in all directions, whereas the processes of the latter are usually aligned perpendicularly to the axon bundles.

Microglial cells are equipped with numerous receptors and immune molecule recognition sites, which make them perfect sensors of the status of the CNS tissue; brain injury is immediately sensed, which initiates the process of activation of microglia. This process turns microglia into an activated (or reactive) state; and some of the activated cells proceed further to become phagocytes. Both reactive microglia and phagocytes provide an active brain defence system (see Chapter 9).

4

Glial Development

4.1 Phylogeny of glia and evolutionary specificity of glial cells in human brain

Glia appear early in phylogeny; even primitive nervous systems of invertebrates such as annelids and leeches, crustacea and insects, and molluscs and cephalopods contain clearly identifiable glial cells, and their study has provided a significant contribution to our understanding of glial cell physiology. Most strikingly, however, the evolution of the CNS is associated with a remarkable increase in the number and complexity of glial cells (Figure 4.1). In the leech, for example, the nervous system is organized in ganglia; each ganglion contains 20–30 neurones, which are coupled to one giant (up to 1 mm in diameter) glial cell. The nervous system of the nematode *Caenorhabditis elegans* contains 302 neurones and only 56 glial cells (i.e. glia account for about 16 per cent of all neural cells). In drosophila, glial cells already account for ~20–25 per cent of cells in the nervous system, and in rodents about 60 per cent of all neural cells are glia.

In human brain, glial cells are certainly the most numerous as it is generally believed that glial cells outnumber neurones in human brain by a factor of 10 to 50; although the precise number of cells in the brain of *Homo sapiens* remains unknown. Early estimates put a total number of neurones at ~85 billion; however, now we know that this number should be substantially larger as a cerebellum alone contains ~105 billion neurones. Therefore, the human brain as a whole may contain several hundred billions of neurones and probably several trillions (or thousand billions) of astrocytes. Morphological data for the cortex are more reliable and they show that human brain has the highest glia to neurone ratio among all species (this ratio is 0.3:1 in mice and about 1.65:1 in human brain – see Figure 4.1). Interestingly, however, the overall volume of the glial compartment remains more or less constant as they occupy about 50 per cent of the nervous system throughout the evolutionary ladder.

Not only does the human brain have the largest number of glia, but the glial cells in primates also show remarkable differences compared to nonprimates. The

Glial Neurobiology: A Textbook   Alexei Verkhratsky and Arthur Butt
© 2007 John Wiley & Sons, Ltd   ISBN 978-0-470-01564-3 (HB); 978-0-470-51740-6 (PB)

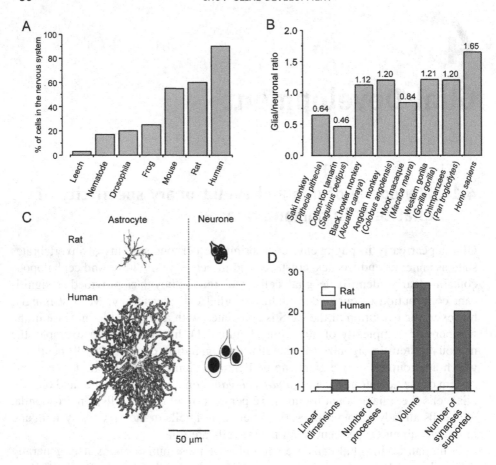

Figure 4.1 Phylogenetical advance of glial cells:

A. Percentage of glial cells is increased in phylogenesis. In fact the total quantity of neural cells in the brain of higher primates, including *Homo sapiens*, is not known precisely; the number of neurones in human brain can be as high as several hundred of billions. It is commonly assumed that glia outnumber neurones in human brain by a factor of 10 to 50 (e.g. Kandel, Nerve cells and behaviour. In: *Principles of neural science*, Kandel ER, Schwartz JH, Jessell TM, Eds, 4th edition, pp. 19–35. New York: McGraw-Hill) although the precise ratio remains to be determined.

B. The numbers of glia and neurones in cortex is more precisely quantified, and this graph shows the glia/neurone ratio in cortex of high primates; this ratio is the highest in humans. (Data are taken from Sherwood CC, Stimpson CD, Raghanti MA, Wildman DE, Uddin M, Grossman LI, Goodman M, Redmond JC, Bonar CJ, Erwin JM, Hof PR (2006) Evolution of increased glia–neuron ratios in the human frontal cortex. *Proc Natl Acad Sci U S A* **103**, 13606–13611).

C. Graphic representation of neurones and astroglia in mouse and in human cortex. Evolution has resulted in dramatic changes in astrocytic dimensions and complexity.

D. Relative increase in glial dimensions and complexity during evolution. Linear dimensions of human astrocytes when compared with mice are ~2.75 times larger; and their volume is 27 times larger; human astrocytes have ~10 times more processes and every astrocyte in human cortex enwraps ~20 times more synapses.

(C, D – adapted from Oberheim NA, Wang X, Goldman S, Nedergaard M (2006) Astrocytic complexity distinguishes the human brain. *Trends Neurosci* **29**, 547–553)

most abundant astroglial cell in human and primate brain are the protoplasmic astrocytes, which densely populate cortex and hippocampus. Human protoplasmic astrocytes are much larger and far more complex than protoplasmic astrocytes in rodent brain. The linear dimensions of human protoplasmic astroglial cells are about 2.75 times larger and have a volume about 27 times greater than the same cells in mouse brain. Furthermore, human protoplasmic astrocytes have about 40 main processes and these processes have immensely more complex branching than mouse astrocytes (which bear only 3–4 main processes). As a result, every human protoplasmic astrocyte contacts and enwraps ~ two million synapses compared to only 90 000 synapses covered by the processes of a mouse astrocyte.

Moreover, the brain of primates contains specific astroglial cells, which are absent in other vertebrates (Figure 4.2). Most notable of these are the interlaminar astrocytes, which reside in layer I of the cortex; this layer is densely populated by synapses but almost completely devoid of neuronal cell bodies. These interlaminar astrocytes have a small cell body (~10 μm), several short and one or two very long processes; the latter penetrate through the cortex, and end in layers III and IV; these processes can be up to 1 mm long. The endings of the long processes create a rather unusual terminal structure, known as the 'terminal mass' or 'end bulb', which are composed of multilaminal structures, containing mitochondria. Most amazingly, the processes of interlaminar astrocytes and size of 'terminal masses' were particularly large in the brain of Albert Einstein; although whether these features were responsible for his genius is not really proven. The function of these interlaminar astrocytes remain completely unknown, although it has been speculated that they are the astroglial counterpart of neuronal columns, which are the functional units of the cortex, and may be responsible for a long-distance signalling and integration within cortical columns. Quite interestingly, interlaminar astrocytes are altered in Down syndrome and Alzheimer's disease.

Human brain also contains polarized astrocytes, which are uni- or bipolar cells which dwell in layers V and VI of the cortex, quite near to the white matter; they have one or two very long (up to 1 mm) processes that terminate in the neuropil. The processes of these cells are thin (2–3 μm in diameter) and straight; they also have numerous varicosities. Once more, the function of polarized astrocytes remains enigmatic; although they might be involved in para-neuronal long-distance signalling.

Most interestingly, the evolution of neurones produced fewer changes in their appearance. That is, the density of synaptic contacts in rodents and primates is very similar (in rodent brain the mean density of synaptic contacts is ~1397 millions/mm^3, which is not very much different from humans – synaptic density in human cortex is around 1100 millions/mm^3). Similarly, the number of synapses per neurone does not differ significantly between primates and rodents. The shape and dimensions of neurones also has not changed dramatically over the phylogenetic ladder: human neurones are certainly larger, yet their linear dimensions are only ~1.5 times greater than in rodents.

Thus, at least morphologically, evolution resulted in far greater changes in glia than in neurones, which most likely has important, although yet undetermined, significance.

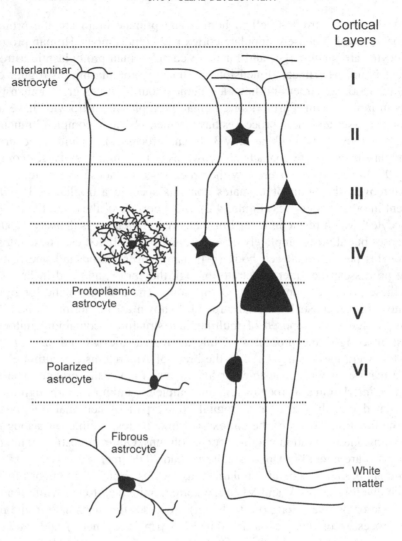

Figure 4.2 Astrocytes of human cortex. Schematic representation of human cortical layers, I to VI. Primate-specific astrocytes are (1) the interlaminar astrocytes, somatas of which reside in Layer I, and processes extend towards layers III and IV, and (2) polarized astrocytes, which are localized in layers V and VI and also send long processes through the cortical layers. Human protoplasmic astrocytes are characterized by a very high complexity of their processes. White matter contains fibrous astrocytes, which are least different from nonprimates. (Modified from Oberheim NA, Wang X, Goldman S, Nedergaard M (2006) Astrocytic complexity distinguishes the human brain. *Trends Neurosci* **29**, 547–553)

4.2 Macroglial cells

All neural cells (i.e. neurones and macroglia) derive from the neuroepithelium, which forms the neural tube. These cells are pluripotent in a sense that their progeny may differentiate into neurones or macroglial cells with equal probability, and therefore these *neuroepithelial cells* may be defined as true '*neural progenitors*'. These neural progenitors give rise to neuronal or glial precursor cells ('neuroblasts' and 'glioblasts', respectively), which in turn differentiate into neurones or macroglial cells. For many years it was believed that the neuroblasts and glioblasts appear very early in development, and that they form two distinct and noninterchangeable pools committed, respectively, to produce strictly neuronal or strictly glial lineages. It was also taken more or less for granted that the pool of precursor cells is fully depleted around birth, and neurogenesis is totally absent in the mature brain.

Recently, however, this paradigm has been challenged, as it appears that neuronal and glial lineages are much more closely related than was previously thought, and that the mature brain still has numerous stem cells, which may provide for neuronal replacement. Moreover, it turns out that neural stem cells have many properties of astroglia.

The modern scheme of neural cell development is illustrated in Figure 4.3 and is as follows: At the origin of all neural cell lineages lie neural progenitors

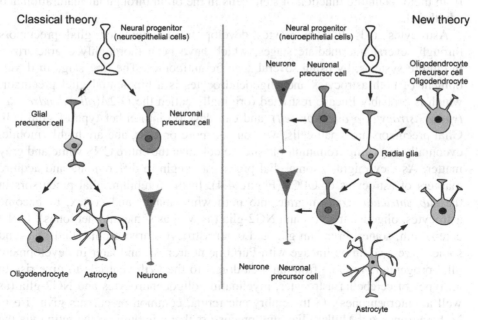

Neural cells lineages

Figure 4.3 Modern views on pathways of neural cell development. Classical theory postulates the very early separation of neural and glial lineages, whereby neural and glial precursors are completely committed to the development of the respective cells (lineage restricted). Recent evidence, however, supports a new hypothesis, in which radial glial cells are multipotent neural precursors, generating neurones and oligodendrocytes, and eventually transforming into astrocytes. Furthermore, radial glia generate a subpopulation of 'stem' neural cells that have properties of astrocytes. These 'stem' astrocytes underlie adult neurogenesis and can produce either neurones or macroglial cells (see the text for further explanation)

in the form of neuroepithelial cells. Morphologically, neural progenitors appear as elongated cells extending between the two surfaces (ventricular and pial) of the neuronal tube. Very early in development, the neural progenitors give rise to *radial glial cells*, which are in fact the first cells that can be distinguished from neuroepithelial cells. The somatas of radial glial cells are located in the *ventricular zone* and their processes extend to the pia. These radial glial cells are the central element in subsequent neurogenesis, because they act as the main neural progenitors during development, giving rise to neurones, astrocytes, and some oligodendrocytes. The majority of oligodendrocytes, however, originate from glial precursors that are generated in specific sites in the brain and spinal cord (see below). Astrocytes are generated both from radial glia and later in development from glial precursors that also give rise to oligodendrocytes; the proportion of the final population of astrocytes derived from radial glia and glial precursors depends on the region of the CNS (see below). Radial glia not only produce neurones, but they also form a scaffold along which newborn neurones migrate from the ventricular zone to their final destinations (see Chapter 7). Moreover, the radial glial cells and astrocytes that differentiate from them retain the function of stem cells in the brain throughout maturation and adulthood.

Astrocytes and oligodendrocytes develop from committed glial precursors through several intermediate stages, which have been thoroughly characterized in culture systems, by using several specific antibodies. The first stage in development of both astrocytes and oligodendrocytes is a bipotential glial precursor, which is probably lineage restricted (originally called the *O-2A(oligodendrocyte-type 2 astrocyte) progenitor cell*), and can develop into either type of glial cell. Glial precursors are small cells, with one or more process, and are highly mobile, eventually migrating from multiple sites to colonize the entire CNS white and grey matter. As they migrate, some glial precursors begin to differentiate and acquire markers of astrocytes or OPCs (Figure 4.4). In the forebrain, glial precursors in the *subventricular zone* migrate into both white matter and cortex, to become astrocytes, oligodendrocytes and NG2-glia (as well as some interneurones). In the cerebellum, some Bergmann glia and other astrocytes arise from radial glia (and some share a common lineage with Purkinje neurones), and later in development glial progenitors migrate from an area dorsal to the IVth ventricle to give rise to all types of cerebellar astrocytes, myelinating oligodendrocytes and NG2-glia (as well as interneurones). In the embryonic retina, common precursors give rise to both neurones and Müller glia; glial precursors that migrate into the retina via the optic nerve give rise to astrocytes, but oligodendrocytes and NG2-glia are absent from the retina of most species. Astrocytes and oligodendrocytes in the spinal cord appear to arise from different precursors in separate areas of the ventricular zone. The ventral neuroepithelium of the embryonic cord is divided into a number of domains, which contain precursors that first generate neurones (motor neurones and interneurones) and then oligodendrocytes. Astrocytes most likely arise from radial glia.

Oligodendroglial lineage

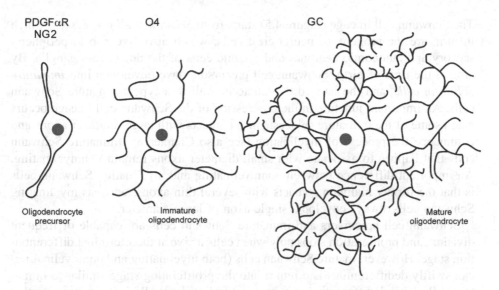

Figure 4.4 Oligodendroglial lineage. Oligodendrocyte precursor cells (OPCs), in culture at least, can generate oligodendrocytes or astrocytes (O-2A cell), although *in vivo* they may only generate oligodendrocytes. OPCs are characterized by expression of platelet-derived growth factor alpha receptors (PDGFαR), the NG2 chondroitin sulphate proteoglycan (SPG), and the ganglioside GD3; these play important roles in proliferation and migration of OPCs. OPCs are generated in localized sources in the brain and spinal cord from which they migrate to their final locations throughout the CNS. There, oligodendrocyte precursors transform into fully committed immature oligodendrocytes, characterized by expression of the O4 antigen. These O4-positive cells further differentiate into mature oligodendrocytes, expressing galactocerebroside (GC) and producing myelin. Under appropriate culture conditions, OPCs spontaneously transform into oligodendrocytes in the absence of axons, but *in vivo* oligodendrocyte proliferation, survival, differentiation and myelination are regulated by axonal signals

4.3 Astroglial cells are brain stem cells

Neurogenesis in the mammalian brain occurs throughout the lifespan. New neurones that continuously appear in the adult brain are added to neural circuits, and may even be responsible for the considerable plasticity of the latter. The appearance of new neurones does not happen in all brain regions of mammals; it is mainly restricted to hippocampus and olfactory bulb (although in nonmammalian vertebrates neurogenesis occurs in almost every brain region).

In both hippocampus (in its subgranular zone) and in the subventricular zone (the latter produces neurones for the olfactory bulb) the stem cells have been identified as astrocytes. It remains unclear whether astroglial cells in other brain regions may also retain these stem cell capabilities.

4.4 Schwann cell lineage

The Schwann cell lineage (Figure 4.5) starts from *Schwann cell precursors*, which in turn, are the progeny of neural crest cells, which also give rise to peripheral sensory and autonomic neurones and satellite cells of the dorsal root ganglia. By around the time of birth, Schwann cell precursors have developed into *immature Schwann cells*, and the latter differentiate into all four types of mature Schwann cells. An important juncture in the progression of the Schwann cell lineage occurs when some of the immature cells establish contacts with large-diameter axons and commence the process of myelination (see also Chapter 8). Immature Schwann cells that happen to associate with small diameter axons remain nonmyelinating. An important difference between nonmyelinating and myelinating Schwann cells is that the former maintain contacts with several thin axons, whereas myelinating Schwann cells always envelop a single axon of large diameter.

Schwann cell precursors and immature Schwann cells are capable of frequent division, and proliferation stops only when cells arrive at their terminal differentiation stage. However, mature Schwann cells (both myelinating and nonmyelinating) can swiftly dedifferentiate and return into the proliferating stage similar to immature cells. This dedifferentiation process underlies the Wallerian degeneration that

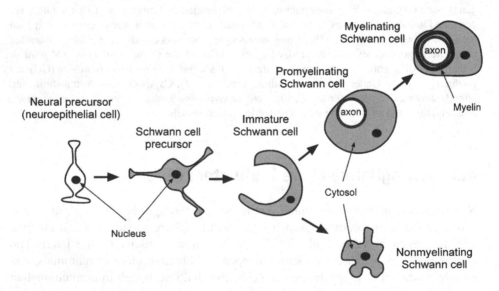

Figure 4.5 Schwann cell lineage. Schwann cell precursors appear from neuroepithelial cells, and differentiate into immature Schwann cells. The latter can further differentiate into either nonmyelinating Schwann cells, or after contacting the axon, transform into pro-myelinating Schwann cells and then myelinating Schwann cells. The differentiation and fate of Schwann cells are under the tight control of axonal signals

follows injury of peripheral nerves (see Chapters 9 and 10). After completion of nerve regeneration, Schwann cells once more redifferentiate.

4.5 Microglial cell lineage

Microglial cells derive from the myelomonocytic lineage, which in turn develops from hemangioblastic mesoderm. The progenitors of microglial cells, known as *foetal macrophages* (Figure 4.6) enter the neural tube at early embryonic stages (e.g. at embryonic day 8 in rodents). These foetal macrophages are tiny rounded cells and in the course of development they transform into embryonic microglia

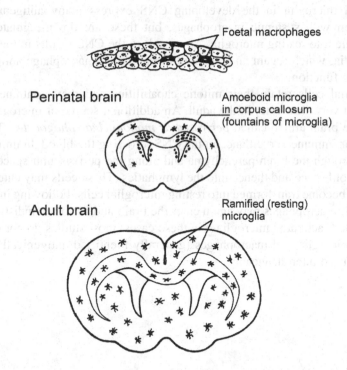

Figure 4.6 Ontogenetic development of microglia. The ontogenetic development of microglia comprises three developmental stages. Foetal macrophages are identified in the neuroepithelium at a very early stage (~8 embryonic day in rodents). In perinatal brain, macrophages invade corpus callosum and form clusters of amoeboid microglia. These amoeboid microglial cells migrate into the brain and transform into ramified, resting microglia. (From W.J. Streit, 'Microglial cells'; In: *Neuroglia*, H. Kettenmann and B.R. Ransom, Eds, 2005, p. 61 by permission of Oxford University Press)

that have a small cell body and several short processes. In the perinatal period, some of microglial precursors turn into *amoeboid microglia*, dense clusters of which appear in the corpus callosum. Del Rio Hortega called these groups of rapidly dividing glial precursors *fountains of microglia*, which persist in the corpus callosum for about two weeks after birth (Figure 4.6). The amoeboid microglial cells proliferate very rapidly and migrate into the cortex, where they settle and turn into *ramified resting microglia*. Microglia play an essential phagocytic role during development, removing the debris that arises from the large degree of neural apoptosis during development. Microglia can be 'killers' as well as 'cleaners' in the developing CNS; for example, in the embryonic retina, immature neurones express receptors for nerve growth factor (NGF) and these are down-regulated as neurones mature, but excess neurones do not lose their receptors and die by apoptosis in response to NGF released by microglia. Microglia are also responsible for immune tolerance to CNS antigens, by migrating into the embryonic CNS and providing a memory of 'self' before the blood–brain barrier is formed, after which the CNS becomes immune privileged and largely isolated from the systemic immune system. Amoeboid microglia in the developing CNS express many antigenic markers in common with systemic macrophages, but these are down-regulated as they differentiate into resting microglia. Any insult to the CNS results in the activation of microglia, which regain an amoeboid morphology, macrophage antigens and a phagocytic function.

Microglial cells retain their mitotic capabilities and they continue to divide (albeit at a very slow rate) in the adult. An additional source of microglial cells in the mature brain are so-called *perivascular mononuclear phagocytes*. These cells provide for immune surveillance in the CNS, crossing the blood–brain barrier and passing through the brain parenchyma and along the perivascular spaces, into the subarachnoid space and thence into the lymphatics. These cells may enter the brain tissue and become transformed into resting microglial cells. Following insults to the adult CNS, macrophages may again enter the brain and are often indistinguishable from resident activated microglia – in these cases, most studies do not distinguish between microglia and macrophages (generally identified antigenically), and the terms are used interchangeably.

5
General Physiology of Glial Cells

5.1 Membrane potential and ion distribution

In general, mature macroglial cells have a negative resting membrane potential ($\sim$ –80 to –90 mV), because of the predominance of potassium conductance, which maintains the membrane potential close to the potassium equilibrium potential (E_K); however, astrocytes are heterogeneous with respect to membrane potentials and potassium conductances, and the 'text-book' view of astrocytes as a homogeneous population of cells with a highly negative membrane potential close to the E_K is an oversimplification (see below). Electrical depolarization of glia results in electrotonic changes of the membrane potential and does not produce regenerative action potentials. The ion distribution across glial membranes is similar to other cells (intracellular K^+ concentration is $\sim$100–140 mM; $Na^+ < 10$ mM, $Ca^{2+} < 0.0001$ mM). The main exception is Cl^-, which is unusually high in both astrocytes and oligodendrocytes ($[Cl^-]_i \sim 30$–40 mM), due to the high activity of $Na^+/K^+/2Cl^-$ cotransporters, which transport $2Cl^-$ into the cell in exchange for 1 K^+ and 1 Na^+.

5.2 Ion channels

Glial cells express all major types of voltage-gated ion channels, including K^+, Na^+ and Ca^{2+}, and various types of anion channels (Table 5.1). Biophysically these channels are similar to those found in other types of cells such as nerve or muscle cells.

Potassium voltage-gated channels are most abundantly present in various types of neuroglia. These channels are represented by four families, known as the *inward rectifier K^+ channels* (K_{ir}), *delayed rectifier potassium channels* (K_D), *rapidly inactivating A-type channels* (K_A) and *calcium-activated K^+ channels* (K_{Ca}).

Inward rectifier potassium channels are present in practically all mature neuroglial cells and are responsible for their very negative (–80 to –90 mV) resting

Glial Neurobiology: A Textbook   Alexei Verkhratsky and Arthur Butt
© 2007 John Wiley & Sons, Ltd   ISBN 978-0-470-01564-3 (HB); 978-0-470-51740-6 (PB)

Table 5.1 Ion channels in glial cells

Ion channel	Molecular identity	Localization	Main function
Calcium channels	Ca_V	Immature astrocytes and oligodendrocytes	Generation of Ca^{2+} signals
Sodium channels	Na_V	Astroglial precursors; cells of glia-derived tumours	Regulation of proliferation (?)
Delayed rectifier potassium channels Ca^{2+}-dependent K+ channels 2-Pore-domain K^+ channels	K_D, K_A K_{Ca} K_V1.4, 1.5 TREK/TASK	Ubiquitous	Maintenance of resting membrane potential; glial proliferation and reactivity
Inward rectifier potassium channels	K_{ir}4.1 (predominant) K_{ir} 2.1, 2.2, 2.3 K_{ir} 3.1 K_{ir} 6.1, 6.2	Ubiquitous	Maintenance of resting membrane potential K^+ buffering
Chloride channels	?	Ubiquitous	Chloride transport; regulation of cell volume
Aquaporins (water channels)	AQP4 (predominant) AQP9	AQP4 – ubiquitous AQP9 – astrocytes in brain stem; ependymal cells; tanycytes in hypothalamus and in subfornical organ	Water transport

membrane potential. They are called inwardly (or anomalously) rectifying because of their peculiar voltage-dependence: these channels tend to be closed when the membrane is depolarized and are activated when the membrane is hyperpolarized to the levels around or more negative than the E_K. In other words, these channels favour potassium diffusion in the inward direction over the outward one. These channels set the resting membrane potential; the K_{ir} channels are regulated by extracellular K^+ concentration, and increases in the latter result in inward flow of K^+ ions, which is important for K^+ removal from the extracellular space, considered a primary physiological function of astrocytes (see Chapter 7).

Molecularly, there are more than 20 types of inwardly rectifying K^+ channels (or K_{ir} channels), and glia express representatives of most kinds. Glia (astrocytes, oligodendrocytes, Müller glia and Bergmann glia) are characterized by expression of the K_{ir}4.1 subtype, which is almost exclusively glial in the CNS, and a critical role for K_{ir}4.1 in setting the negative glial membrane potential has been demonstrated in K_{ir}4.1 knockout mice. In addition to K_{ir}4.1, glia express diverse K_{ir}, including: K_{ir}5.1, which do not form functional homomeric channels, but form heteromeric channels by a specific coassembly with K_{ir}4.1; members of the strongly rectifying and constitutively active K_{ir} 2.0 family (e.g. K_{ir}2.1, 2.2 and 2.3), which may also specifically coassemble with K_{ir}4.1 in glia; K_{ir}3.0 channels (e.g. K_{ir}3.1), which are coupled to a range of G-protein linked neurotransmitter receptors (K_{ir}3.0 channels are generally formed by coassembly of K_{ir}3.1 subunits with other members of the same family, such as the K_{ir}3.1/K_{ir}3.4 heteromers in atrial myocytes, which are responsible for the acetylcholine (ACh)-induced deceleration of heart beat); and ATP-dependent K_{ir} (K_{ir}6.1 and 6.2), which are only active when intracellular concentrations of ATP fall to very low levels and therefore serve to maintain the high K^+ conductance and hyperpolarized resting membrane potential in glia during metabolic challenge. Glia also express two-pore domain K^+ (2PK) channels, which are responsible for the background or leak K^+ conductance and are involved in setting the resting membrane potential and ion and water homeostasis; glia express TREK and TASK subtypes of 2PK channels.

Delayed rectifier potassium channels, rapidly inactivating A-type channels, and calcium-dependent channels   are expressed in practically every type of glial cell. Molecularly, glial cells express multiple K_D channel subtypes, but apparently only one K_A channel subtype, K_v1.4, which may form heteromers with the K_D channel subunit K_v1.5. Three types of K_{Ca} can be distinguished by their biophysical properties (BK, IK and SK), and glia express both BK and SK; BK channels are strongly voltage-dependent and sensitive to micromolar calcium, whereas SK are weakly voltage-dependent and sensitive to nanomolar calcium. K_D, K_A and K_{Ca} are all closed at the resting membrane potential and their activation requires depolarization of the cell membrane to values more positive than -40 mV. Hence, the functional role of these channels in glial cells remains unclear. However, they may be activated when extracellular potassium concentration is elevated sufficiently to depolarize the cell membrane; for example, Kv1.5 and BK channels are localized to Schwann cell membranes at nodes of Ranvier, where localized increases in K^+ and Ca^{2+} during action potential propagation may be sufficient for them to open, and the consequent K^+ efflux may play a role in the post-stimulus recovery of extracellular potassium levels. Although the function of K_D in mature glia is unclear, they are important for glial proliferation during development and following CNS injury.

Voltage-gated sodium channels (Na_V)   are found in many types of astroglial cells, including retinal astrocytes, astrocytes from hippocampus, cortex and spinal cord, and in Schwann cells. The molecular structure and biophysical properties of Na_V channels expressed in glial cells are similar to those present in neurones or muscle cells. The main difference is the channel density: glial cells have about one Na_V channel per 10 μm^2, whereas their density in neurones can reach 1000– 10 000 per 1 μm^2. The role of Na_V channels in glia remains unclear; interestingly glial progenitor cells may have a much higher density of Na_V, similarly very high densities of Na_V were found in tumours of glial origin, and it may be that

Na_V channels are somehow involved in the control of glial cell proliferation, differentiation or migration.

Voltage-gated calcium channels (Ca_V)   are usually detected in glial precursors or in immature glial cells, and may be important for generating local elevations in cytosolic calcium concentration relevant for controlling growth or migration of neuroglial precursors. Current evidence is that Ca_V are down-regulated during glial development, but they are up-regulated in reactive astrocytes, consistent with a role for Ca_V in proliferation and growth. The localization of Ca_V to the processes of immature oligodendrocytes suggests a role in myelination. Müller glia express mRNA for Ca_V subunits, and astrocytes and myelinating oligodendrocytes may express voltage-gated calcium channels in microdomains. The expression of Ca_V by mature glia remains uncertain, because of the inability of patch-clamp and calcium-imaging techniques to identify small currents or calcium signals that may occur at distal processes.

Chloride and other anion channels   several types have been demonstrated in astrocytes, oligodendrocytes and Schwann cells. Importantly, astrocytes are able to actively accumulate Cl^-, resulting in a relatively high intracellular Cl^- concentration (about 35 mM), largely through the activity of $Na^+/K^+/Cl^-$ cotransporters. The equilibrium potential for Cl^- in astrocytes lies around –40 mV, and therefore opening of Cl^--selective channels leads to Cl^- efflux (manifested electrically as an inward current depolarizing the cells, because of loss of anions). The Cl^- channels may be involved in astrocyte swelling and in the regulation of extracellular Cl^- concentration.

Aquaporins   are integral membrane proteins, which form channels permeable to water and to some other molecules e.g. glycerol and urea. There are at least 10 different types of aquaporins (AQP1 to AQP10) in mammalian cells, and AQP4 is expressed almost exclusively by astrocytes throughout the brain; in addition astrocytes also have small amounts of AQP9. Aquaporins are concentrated on astroglial perivascular endfeet, where they are colocalized with $K_{ir}4.1$; they may be particularly important during cerebral oedema, when astroglial perivascular endfeet swell considerably and protect the surrounding neurones. In the hypothalamus and in osmosensory areas of the subfornical organ, tanycytes exclusively express AQP9 (and they do not possess AQP4), which may be involved in regulation of systemic water homeostasis.

5.3   Receptors to neurotransmitters and neuromodulators

Glial cells are capable of expressing the same extended variety of receptors as neurones do, which allows glia to actively sense information delivered by neurotransmitters released during synaptic transmission. Glia, similar to neurones, are endowed with both ionotropic and metabotropic receptors, and the main classes of glial neurotransmitter receptors are summarized in Table 5.2.

Initial experiments on astroglial cells isolated from the brain and grown in culture demonstrated that these cells are capable of expressing almost all types of neurotransmitter receptor (Figure 5.1), and moreover different cells may have quite

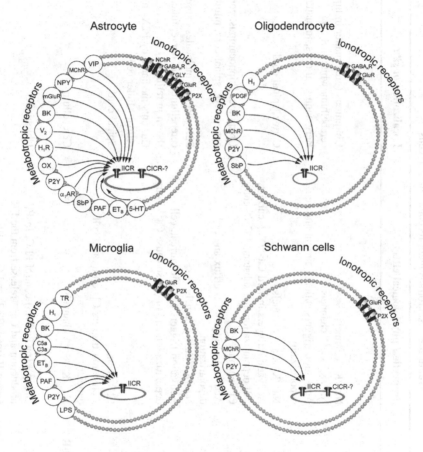

Figure 5.1 Neurotransmitter receptors in glial cells – scheme showing the multiplicity of neurotransmitter receptors expressed in different types of glial cells. IICR – InsP3-induced Ca^{2+}release; CICR – Ca^{2+}-induced Ca^{2+} release.

Ionotropic receptors: NChr – Nicotinic Cholinoreceptors; $GABA_A R$ – GABA receptors; GLY – glycine receptors; GluR – glutamate receptors (AMPA, NMDA and KA receptors); P2X – purinoreceptors.

Metabotropic receptors: VIP – vasoactive intestinal polypeptide receptors; MChR – muscarinic cholinoreceptors; NPY – neuropeptide Y receptors; mGluR – metabotropic glutamate receptors; BK – bradykinin receptors; V2 – vasopressin receptors; $H_1 R$ – histamine receptors; OX – oxytocin receptors; P2Y – metabotropic purinoreceptors; $\alpha_1 AR$ – adrenergic receptors; SbP – substance P receptors; PAF – platelet activating factor receptors; ET_B – endothelin receptors; 5-HT – serotonin receptors

Table 5.2 Neurotransmitter receptors in glial cells

Receptor type	Properties/ physiological effect	Localization *in situ*
Astrocytes		
Ionotropic receptors		
A. Glutamate receptors	Na^+/K^+ channels	Ubiquitous (grey matter in hippocampus, cortex,
AMPA/Kainate	$Na^+/K^+/Ca^{2+}$ channels	cerebellum, white matter)
	Activation triggers cationic current and cell depolarization	Bergmann glial cells, immature astrocytes
NMDA receptors	$Na^+/K^+/Ca^{2+}$ channels	Cortex, spinal cord
	Activation triggers inward Ca^{2+}/Na^+ current, cell depolarization and substantial Ca^{2+} entry	
B. GABA$_A$ receptors	Cl^- channel	Ubiquitous (hippocampus, cortex, cerebellum,
	Activation triggers Cl- efflux and cell depolarization	optic nerve, spinal cord, pituitary gland)
C. P2X (ATP) Purinoreceptors	$Na^+/K^+/Ca^{2+}$ channels	P2X receptor molecules expressed in cortex,
	Activation triggers cationic current, cell depolarization and may also cause Ca^{2+} entry	cerebellum, optic nerve; functional activation shown in retina
		Currents mediated by P2X$_7$ receptors are found in retinal Müller cells
D. Glycine receptors	Cl^- channel	Spinal cord
	Activation triggers Cl- efflux and cell depolarization	
E. Nicotinic cholinoreceptors NChR	$Na^+/K^+/Ca^{2+}$ channels	Cerebellum
Metabotropic receptors		
A. Glutamate receptors (mGluRs)	Group I (mGluR1,5) control PLC, InsP$_3$ production and Ca^{2+} release from the ER Group II (mGluR2,3) and Group III (mGluR4,6,7) control synthesis of cAMP	Ubiquitous

B. GABA$_B$ receptors	Control PLC, InsP$_3$ production and Ca^{2+} release from the ER	Hippocampus
C. Adenosine receptors A$_1$, A$_2$, A$_3$	A$_1$ receptors control PLC, InsP$_3$ production and Ca^{2+} release from the ER A$_2$ receptor increase cAMP	Hippocampus, cortex
D. P2Y (ATP) Purinoreceptors	Control PLC, InsP$_3$ production and Ca^{2+} release from the ER	Ubiquitous
E. Adrenergic receptors α_1AR, α_2AR	Control PLC, InsP$_3$ production and Ca^{2+} release from the ER	Hippocampus, Bergmann glial cells Cortex, optic nerve
β_1AR, β_1AR	Control glial cell proliferation and astrogliosis; β_2AR are up-regulated in pathology	
F. Muscarinic cholinoreceptors mChR M$_1$–M$_5$	Control PLC, InsP$_3$ production and Ca^{2+} release from the ER	Hippocampus, amygdala
G. Oxytocin and vasopressin receptors	Control PLC, InsP$_3$ production and Ca^{2+} release from the ER; may regulate water channel (aquaporin)	Hypothalamus, other brain regions(?)
H. Vasoactive Intestinal Polypeptide receptors (VIPR 1,2,3)	Control PLC, InsP$_3$ production and Ca^{2+} release from the ER; may regulate energy metabolism, expression of glutamate transporters, induce release of cytokines and promote proliferation	Supraoptic nucleus; other brain regions(?)
I. Serotonin receptors 5-HT$_{1A}$, 5-HT$_{2A}$, 5-HT$_{5A}$	Increase in cAMP, energy metabolism	?
J. Angiotentsin receptors AT$_1$, AT$_2$	Control PLC, InsP$_3$ production and Ca^{2+} release from the ER	White matter (optic nerve, corpus callosum, white mater tracts in cerebellum and subcortical areas)
K. Bradykinin receptors B$_1$, B$_2$	Control PLC, InsP$_3$ production and Ca^{2+} release from the ER	?

Table 5.2   (Continued)

Receptor type	Properties/ physiological effect	Localization *in situ*
L. Thyrotropic-releasing hormone receptors, TRH$_1$	?	Spinal cord
M. Opioid receptors, μ, δ, κ	Inhibition of DNA synthesis, proliferation and growth, inhibition of cAMP production	Hippocampus
N. Histamine receptors, H$_1$	Control PLC, InsP$_3$ production and Ca^{2+} release from the ER	Hippocampus, cerebellum
H$_2$	Control synthesis of cAMP	
O. Dopamine receptors D$_1$	Control synthesis of cAMP	Cortex
D$_2$	Trigger Ca^{2+} signals	
Oligodendrocytes *Ionotropic receptors*		
A. Glutamate receptors AMPA/Kainate	Na$^+$/K$^+$ (Ca^{2+}) channels Activation triggers cationic current and cell depolarization	Corpus callosum, spinal cord, optic nerve
NMDA	Ca^{2+}/Na$^+$/K$^+$ channels	Optic nerve, corpus callosum, cerebellar white matter; may be activated upon pathological insult and contribute to oligodendrocyte death
B. GABA$_A$ receptors	Cl$^-$ channel Activation triggers Cl- efflux and cell depolarization	Corpus callosum

Receptor	Function	Location
C. Glycine receptors	Cl^- channel; Activation triggers Cl- efflux and cell depolarization	Spinal cord
Metabotropic receptors		
A. Muscarinic cholinoreceptors mChR M_1, M_2	Control synthesis of cAMP	?
B. P2Y (ATP) Purinoreceptors	Control PLC, $InsP_3$ production and Ca^{2+} release from the ER	Corpus callosum
Microglia		
Ionotropic receptors		
A. P2X (ATP) Purinoreceptors	$Na^+/K^+/Ca^{2+}$ channels; Activation triggers cationic current and cell depolarization; may also cause substantial Ca^{2+} influx	Ubiquitous; specifically important are P2X7 receptors, which trigger release of cytokines. Expression of P2X receptors is modulated by microglial activation
B. Glutamate receptors AMPA/Kainate	Na^+/K^+ channels; Activation triggers cationic current and cell depolarization	?
Metabotropic receptors		
A. P2Y (ATP) Purinoreceptors	Control PLC, $InsP_3$ production and Ca^{2+} release from the ER; Modulate interleukin release	Ubiquitous
B. $GABA_B$ receptors		?
C. Muscarinic cholinergic receptors	Control PLC, $InsP_3$ production and Ca^{2+} release from the ER	Cultures rat and human microglia
D. Cytokine/complement receptors	Control PLC, $InsP_3$ production and Ca^{2+} release from the ER, control energy status, regulate release of pro-inflammatory factors	Ubiquitous

Table 5.2 (Continued)

Receptor type	Properties/ physiological effect	Localization *in situ*
E. Chemokine receptors (CCR1–5, CXCR4 etc.)	Control PLC, $InsP_3$ production and Ca^{2+} release from the ER; may activate JAK/STAT and NF-κB pathways	Ubiquitous
F. Endothelin receptors, ET_B	Control PLC, $InsP_3$ production and Ca^{2+} release from the ER	Ubiquitous
Schwann cells		
Ionotropic receptors		
A. P2X (ATP) Purinoreceptors	$Na^+/K^+/Ca^{2+}$ channels Activation triggers cationic current and cell depolarization; may also cause substantial Ca^{2+} influx	Ubiquitous; $P2X_7$ receptors are particularly strongly expressed
Metabotropic receptors		
A. P2X (ATP) Purinoreceptors	Control PLC, $InsP_3$ production and Ca^{2+} release from the ER	Ubiquitous
B. Endothelin receptors, ET_B	Promote Schwann cells proliferation; may be involved in pain mechanisms	?
C. Tachykinin receptors, NK_1	Control PLC, $InsP_3$ production and Ca^{2+} release from the ER	?

different complements of these receptors. When expression of neurotransmitter receptors was further investigated in *in situ* preparations in brain slices, it turned out that astrocytes in different brain regions express a very distinct and limited set of receptors, specific for neurotransmitters released in their vicinity. For example (Figure 5.2) Bergmann glial cells express receptors that exactly match the modality of receptors expressed by its neuronal neighbour, Purkinje neurone. In both cells, the repertoire of receptors is optimized to sense neurotransmitters released by neuronal afferents, which form synapses on this neurone–glial unit. Receptor expression can be even more spatially segregated: the same Bergmann glial cells specifically concentrate receptors for GABA in the membranes surrounding inhibitory synapses signalling to Purkinje neurones. Therefore, the expression of specific receptors is selectively regulated, which makes astrocytes perceptive towards chemical signals specific for each particular region of the brain. As shown

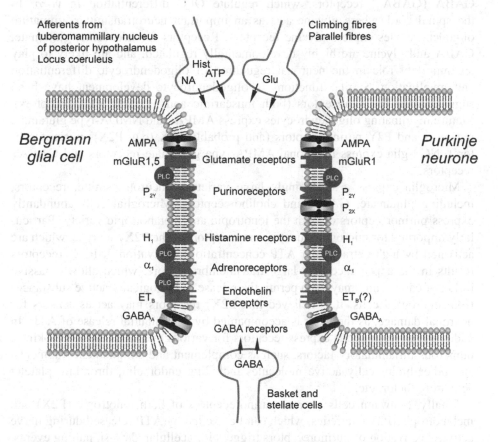

Figure 5.2 Receptors expressed in Bergman glial cell *in situ* are limited to those specific to neurotransmitters released in their vicinity. (Used with permission from Verkhratsky *et al.*, 'Glial calcium: homeostasis and signaling function', *Physiological Reviews*, **78**, 99–141 © 1998)

in Table 5.2, astroglial cells may express a wide variety of receptors; the main types are glutamate receptors, purinoreceptors and GABA receptors. In addition, astrocytes express multiple receptors to neuropeptides, cytokines and chemokines, which are particularly important for regulation of growth and differentiation and for pathological reactions of glial cells.

Oligodendrocytes, in general, express fewer types of neurotransmitter receptors compared to astroglial cells (Table 5.2). Among the most abundant receptors in oligodendrocytes are metabotropic P2Y purinoreceptors, which control cytosolic Ca^{2+} signalling. Immature oligodendrocytes and OPCs also express adenosine (A1) receptors. Oligodendrocytes appear to express ionotropic glutamate receptors of the AMPA/KA kind at all stages of their development, and recent data indicates they also express NMDA receptors. OPCs and immature oligodendrocytes can also express $GABA_A$ receptors, which induce cell depolarization, similar to astrocytes. OPCs also express metabotropic glutamate and GABA ($GABA_B$) receptors, which regulate OPC differentiation *in vitro*. In the spinal cord, where glycine acts as an important neurotransmitter, immature oligodendrocytes express glycine receptors. Receptors for adenosine, glutamate, GABA and glycine are highly developmentally regulated, and are likely to play an important role in the neuronal regulation of oligodendrocyte differentiation and myelination. Similar functions in oligodendrocyte development have been suggested for cholinoreceptors (both muscarinic and nicotinic ACh receptors). Mature myelinating oligodendrocytes express AMPA- and NMDA-type glutamate receptors and P2Y purinoreceptors (and probably P2X (e.g. $P2X_7$) purinoreceptors). NG2-glia express functional AMPA-type glutamate receptors and $GABA_A$ receptors.

Microglia express a surprizingly large variety of neurotransmitter receptors, including glutamate, GABA and cholinoreceptors. Microglial cells abundantly express purinoreceptors of both the ionotropic and metabotropic variety. Particularly important for microglial function are receptors of the $P2X_7$ subtype, which are activated by high extracellular ATP concentrations; activation of $P2X_7$ receptors results in the appearance of a large transmembrane pore, which allows massive influx of cations and may even permit the release of biologically active substances from microglial cells. It is believed that $P2X_7$ receptors may act as sensors for neuronal damage, as the latter is accompanied by a substantial release of ATP. In addition, microglial cells express receptors for various cytokines and chemokines, numerous inflammatory factors, such as complement and complement fragments, and other biologically active molecules including endothelin, thrombin, platelet activating factor, etc.

Finally, Schwann cells express purinoreceptors of both ionotropic (P2X) and metabotropic (P2Y) varieties, which can be excited by ATP released during nerve activity; activation of purinoreceptors triggers intracellular Ca^{2+} signalling events. In addition, Schwann cells are sometimes endowed with endothelin (ET_A and ET_B) receptors and tachykinin receptors of the NK1 type. The ET_A receptors in Schwann cells may be involved in transmission of chronic inflammatory pain.

Below, we shall overview the main types of neurotransmitter receptors expressed in glial cells.

5.3.1 Glutamate receptors

Glutamate is the main excitatory amino acid neurotransmitter in the brain, and glial cells, like neurones, express a wide variety of ionotropic and metabotropic glutamate receptors (Figure 5.3).

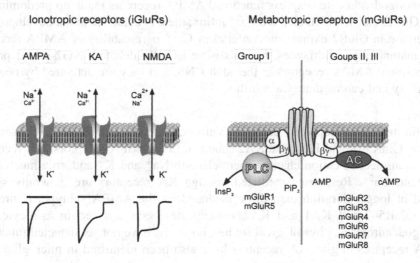

Figure 5.3 Types of glutamate receptors; two fundamentally different classes of glutamate receptors are represented by *ionotropic receptors (iGluR)* and seven-transmembrane-domain G-protein coupled *metabotropic receptors (mGluR)*.

The iGluR are divided into three distinct subtypes, following the discovery of specific pharmacological tools: AMPA (α -amino-3-hydroxy-5-methyl-4-isoxazolepropionic acid), kainate (KA) and NMDA (N-methyl-D-aspartate) receptors. Every subtype of ionotropic glutamate receptor is assembled from four to five specific subunits, which determines receptor functional properties. The AMPA and KA receptors are predominantly permeable to Na^+ and K^+, although they may have Ca^{2+} permeability (maximal P_{Ca}/P_{Na} for AMPA/KA receptors is < 1); NMDA receptors are highly Ca^{2+} permeable ($P_{Ca}/P_{Na} \sim 10-11$). When activated by glutamate, AMPA receptors undergo rapid desensitization (with time constant $\sim$100 ms); KA receptors desensitize slower, and NMDA receptors show almost no desensitization (approximate kinetics of ion current responses to glutamate are shown on the lower panel).

The mGluR mediated intracellular second messenger signalling cascades represented by the InsP3/DAG cascade (mGluRs of Group I, linked to PLC) and cAMP cascade (mGluRs of Groups II and III, linked to AC). The subunits that form the different mGluR are indicated

Ionotropic glutamate receptors (iGluRs)   are abundantly expressed in astroglial cells throughout the CNS. Classically, the iGluRs are subdivided into three major classes, different in molecular structure, pharmacology and biophysical properties. The first class is represented by *AMPA-type receptors*, so called because they are specifically activated by α-amino-3-hydroxy-5-methyl-γ-isoxazolepropionate (AMPA). The AMPA receptors are assembled from four subunits, GluR1 to GluR4, which form cation channels permeable to Na^+ and K^+. When the GluR2 subunit is missing from the assembly, the cation channel is also permeable to Ca^{2+} ions. Glutamate rapidly opens the AMPA receptors, and in the presence of agonist they undergo swift desensitization – i.e. membrane responses mediated through AMPA receptors are fast and are fully inactivated within $\sim$100 ms. AMPA-receptors are present in astroglial cells in most of the brain regions, such as cortex, hippocampus, cerebellum and retina. AMPA receptors are also expressed in astrocytes from corpus callosum and spinal cord and in subpopulations of microglial cells. OPCs and oligodendrocytes express functional AMPA receptors made up predominantly of GluR3 and 4, which mediate Ca^{2+} influx; there is evidence that a developmental increase in GluR2 expression confers low Ca^{2+} permeability of AMPA receptors in mature oligodendrocytes, but this issue is hotly debated. NG2-glia expresses functional AMPA receptors in the adult CNS, and they are activated by neuronal activity and can mediate Ca^{2+} influx.

Kainate (KA)-receptors   are specifically activated by kainate and are assembled from GluR5–7, and KA1 and KA2 subunits. Like AMPA receptors, KA receptors are nonselective cation channels permeable to Na^+ and K^+ and, to a much lesser extent, Ca^{2+}. Responses mediated through KA receptors are generally slower and of longer duration than those mediated by the AMPA subtype. Expression of GluR5–7 and KA1 and KA2 subunits has been detected in astrocytes and oligodendrocytes; physiological studies, however, have not yet detected functional KA receptors in glia. KA receptors have also been identified in microglial cells, but their role remains enigmatic.

NMDA-receptors   – the third type of ionotropic glutamate receptors are specifically activated by N-methyl-D-aspartate (NMDA), and are assembled from several subunits (an NR1 subunit, together with NR2A–NR2D and NR3A–NR3B). NMDA receptors are also cation channels, but differ from other iGluRs in their Ca^{2+} permeability and kinetics. The NMDA receptors are highly permeable for Ca^{2+} (permeability ratio $Ca^{2+}:Na^+$ is $\sim$11:1), and the membrane responses mediated by NMDA receptors are long lasting. Functional NMDA receptors have been demonstrated in astroglial cells in the cortex and spinal cord, and in Müller glia. Recent studies also indicate that NMDA receptors are localized to the myelin sheaths of oligodendrocytes of the optic nerve, corpus callosum and cerebellar white matter. In contrast to neuronal NMDA receptors, glial ones display a weak Mg^{2+} block, and therefore can be activated at the resting membrane potential (in neurones, the ion channel of the NMDA receptor is blocked by Mg^{2+}, which is removed only when the neurone is depolarized, as e.g. following activation of AMPA receptors).

Metabotropic glutamate receptors (mGluRs)   are typical seven-transmembrane-domain (7TM) receptors, which regulate two distinct intracellular signalling pathways (Figure 5.3). The Group I receptors (mGluR 1 and 5) are positively coupled to phospholipase C, and their activation increases the intracellular concentration of $InsP_3$, which subsequently triggers Ca^{2+} release from the endoplasmic reticulum (ER) store. The remaining mGluR subtypes, which belong to Group II (mGluR2, mGluR3) and Group III (mGluR4, mGluR6–8) are coupled to adenylate cyclase and regulate intracellular levels of cAMP. Astroglial cells predominantly express mGluR1, mGluR3 and mGluR5 (i.e. Group I and II); hence glutamate triggers glial Ca^{2+} signals and regulates cAMP-dependent reactions, such as inhibition of K^+ currents, swelling, proliferation and regulation of expression of glutamate transporters. The mGluRs are also present in immature oligodendrocytes and in microglial cells.

5.3.2 Purinoreceptors

The broad class of purinoreceptors are represented by molecules sensing various purinergic nucleotides, which are commonly present in the brain interstitium. These purinergic nucleotides, represented by adenosine triphosphate, adenosine and their metabolites, are released from both neurones and glial cells in several ways. Generally, purinoreceptors are divided into *adenosine (A) receptors* and ATP or *P2 receptors of the P2X (ionotropic) and P2Y (metabotropic) subtypes* (Figure 5.4). All glial cell types have been shown to express adenosine, P2X and P2Y receptors.

All three types of adenosine receptors (of A_1–A_3 types) are expressed in astroglial cells, although their exact role in astrocytes from different brain regions remains mostly unknown; astrocytes release ATP, which is the primary astroglial signalling molecule ('gliotransmitter'), and ATP is rapidly broken down to adenosine, which may serve as a 'gliotransmitter' in some areas. The adenosine receptors are coupled with G-proteins and exert several metabotropic effects. For example, A_1 and A_3 receptors inhibit glial proliferation, whereas A_2 receptors have a stimulatory effect. In addition, stimulation of adenosine receptors may regulate expression of glutamate transporters, sensitivity of cells to glutamate, etc. Adenosine receptors are expressed by OPCs and immature oligodendrocytes, and they mediate axon–glial signalling during myelination. Myelinating and nonmyelinating Schwann cells express adenosine receptors, but they are not involved in axon–glial signalling.

The P2 ATP-receptors (Figure 5.4) are abundantly expressed in all types of glial cells. The expression is particularly prominent for metabotropic P2Y receptors, which are present almost in all types of astrocytes, oligodendrocytes, and microglia throughout the brain and spinal cord, as well as in Schwann cells. These receptors are represented by an extended family ($P2Y_1$ to $P2Y_{14}$); functionally they are

P2 (ATP) Purinoreceptors

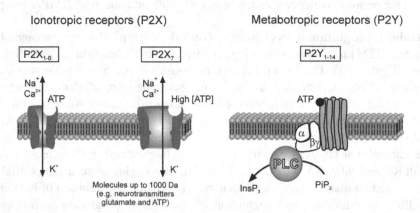

Figure 5.4 P2 (ATP) purinoreceptors are divided into *ionotropic (P2X)* and *metabotropic (P2Y)* receptors.

P2X receptors are ligand-gated cation channels, which upon ATP binding undergo rapid conformational change that allows the passage of Na^+, K^+ and Ca^{2+} through the channel pore (Ca^{2+} permeability relative to monovalent cations can range between 2 and 12 depending on the subunit composition). P2X receptors are formed from seven subunits, $P2X_1$ to $P2X_7$, encoded by distinct genes. The $P2X_{1-6}$ subunits may form homo- or heteromeric receptors, with each functional receptor containing at least three monomers. On activation, $P2X_7$ receptors can form a large pore, which allows passage of molecules with m.w. up to 900–1000 Da; it is generally considered that $P2X_7$ receptors are activated by high concentrations of ATP, and they are particularly important in microglia.

P2Y receptors are classical seven-transmembrane-domain metabotropic receptors coupled to G-proteins. The $P2Y_1$, $P2Y_6$, $P2Y_{11}$, $P2Y_{12}$, $P2Y_{13}$ and $P2Y_{14}$ receptors are detected in the CNS, and all may be expressed in glial cells. Activation of glial P2Y receptors most commonly triggers InsP3-mediated release of Ca^{2+} from endoplasmic reticulum Ca^{2+} stores; $P2Y_1$ receptors are important in astroglial Ca^{2+} signalling

usually positively coupled to phospholipase C (PLC) and their activation triggers cytoplasmic Ca^{2+} signals and intercellular Ca^{2+} waves. The activation of P2Y receptors results in a transient increase in cytosolic Ca^{2+} that can last for seconds to minutes. A special role for the $P2Y_1$ receptor subtype has been indicated in the propagation of astroglial Ca^{2+} waves. Ionotropic ATP receptors of the P2X class have been identified in astrocytes, oligodendrocytes, and in retinal Müller cells *in situ*. P2X receptors are generally rapidly desensitizing and their activation results in a transient ion current (generally inward Na^+ current) lasting milliseconds; their functional role in glia remains undefined. Several types of P2X receptors are expressed in microglial cells; particularly important are $P2X_7$ receptors, which are activated by high (>1 mM) ATP concentrations. Such a high ATP concentration can be achieved during neuronal damage and lysis and therefore $P2X_7$ receptors may enable microglial cells to sense neuronal damage.

Activation of P2X$_7$ receptors results in opening of a large channel, which allows passage of molecules up to 1 kDa; this property is somehow associated with microglial activation. P2X$_7$ receptors play similar roles in pathology in Müller glia, Schwann cells, and oligodendrocytes, and possibly astrocytes. It is not clear that P2X$_7$ receptors form pores in glia, and P2X$_7$ receptors are not the only kinds of P2X receptors expressed by glia that are capable of pore-formation. In astrocytes, P2X$_7$ receptors may mediate the release of ATP.

5.3.3 GABA receptors

The ionotropic γ-aminobutiric acid receptors of *GABA$_A$ type* (Figure 5.5) are expressed by astroglial cells throughout the brain regions, including hippocampus, cerebellum, pituitary gland, optic nerve, retina and spinal cord, and in oligodendrocytes. Molecularly, these receptors are the same as neuronal ones, being in essence ligand-gated Cl$^-$ channels. Functionally, however, there is a remarkable difference, because glial cells contain much more Cl$^-$ than mature neurones (35 mM vs. ~3–5 mM) , and therefore the equilibrium potential for Cl$^-$ in astrocytes and oligodendrocytes is about –40 mV, whereas in neurones it lies somewhere near –70 mV. As a consequence, activation of GABA$_A$ receptors in glial cells triggers efflux of Cl$^-$ ions and cell depolarization. Interestingly, activation of GABA$_A$ receptors also inhibits astroglial K$^+$ channels thus facilitating depolarization.

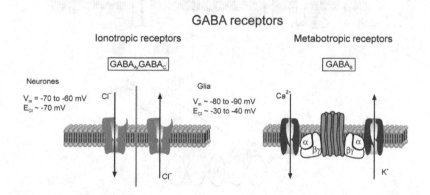

Figure 5.5 GABA receptors are represented by ionotropic GABA$_{A/C}$ receptors and metabotropic GABA$_B$ receptors. GABA$_A$ receptors are ligand gated Cl$^-$ channels, and on their activation Cl$^-$ moves according to the electrochemical gradient; in neurones, the equilibrium potential for Cl$^-$ (E$_{Cl}$) is –70 mV, and activation of GABA$_A$ receptors results in Cl$^-$ influx and hyperpolarization, whereas glia have a strongly negative resting membrane potential (V$_m$) and high intracellular Cl$^-$ concentration (E$_{Cl}$ of –30 to –40 mV), so that activation of GABA$_A$ receptors results in Cl$^-$ efflux and depolarization. GABA$_B$ receptors are coupled to G proteins that control opening of K$^+$ and Ca^{2+} channels

Some astroglial cells (e.g. in hippocampus) and OPCs express metabotropic *GABA$_B$ receptors* coupled with InsP$_3$ metabolism and Ca^{2+} release from the intra-cellular stores.

5.3.4   Cytokine and chemokine receptors

All types of glial cells express various combinations of cytokine and chemokine receptors, which in general control their proliferation, growth and metabolism. These receptors are involved in numerous pathological reactions of glial cells.

The cytokine receptors are represented by two types, type I and type II receptors, which are activated by interferons and interleukins (IL-2, 4, 6, 10, 12, 15 and 21). The signalling pathways triggered by activation of these receptors involve the Janus kinases (JAKs), which in turn control numerous secondary signal transduction proteins, such as for example Signal Transducers and Activators of Transcription (STATs). The latter, after being phosphorylated by JAKs, translocate into the

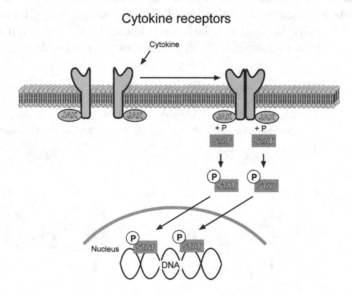

Figure 5.6 Cytokine receptors – there are many, but the most common are associated with the Janus kinase/signal transducer and activator of transcription (JAK/STAT) pathway. Binding of cytokines to the receptor initiates receptor oligomerization and phosphorylation by closely associated JAKs. The phosphorylated receptor becomes a docking site for STAT proteins, which are also phosphorylated by JAKs. Phosphorylated STATs dissociate from the receptors, dimerize and are translocated to the nucleus, where they interact with DNA, hence regulating transcription of genes. (Adapted from Wessman DR, Benveniste EN (2005) Cytokine and chemokine receptors and signaling, In: *Neuroglia*, Kettenmann H & Ransom BR, Eds, OUP, p. 146–162)

nucleus where they initiate transcriptions of various genes, generally known as cytokine responsive genes (Figure 5.6).

The second main signalling pathway controlled by cytokines is represented by tumour necrosis factor (TNF) receptors of the TNFRI and TNFRII families present in all types of glial cells. Activation of TNF receptors regulates activity of JAKs and also utilizes the activation of intracellular transcription factor NF-κB.

Glial cells also express a variety of chemokine receptors. The chemokines are small signalling molecules (8–14 kDa), which regulate cell migration. Chemokine receptors (designated as CCR1–9 and CXCRs) belong to classic seven-transmembrane-domain metabotropic receptors coupled with G-proteins, which in turn, control activation of PLC and phosphatidylinositol-3-OH-kinase (PI3K). Further signalling proceeds through either $InsP_3$, which activates Ca^{2+} release from the ER, or through DAG, which activates protein kinase C (PKC). Activation of chemokine receptors may also activate JAK/STAT and NF-κB pathways. Chemokine receptors are abundantly expressed in microglia, and they are involved in their activation.

5.3.5 Complement receptors

The complement system is one of the key parts of immune response, components of which are also present in the CNS. In particular, the complement anaphylotoxines C3a and C5a are released in the brain at sites of complement activation. Both astrocytes and microglial cells express C3a and C5a receptors, which control Ca^{2+} release from the ER stores via an $InsP_3$-dependent pathway. Expression of C3a and C5a receptors may be up-regulated during inflammation.

5.3.6 Endothelin receptors

Endothelins (ET), which come in three related varieties, ET1 ET2 and ET3, are vasoactive peptides produced mainly by endothelial cells; they can also be produced by astrocytes. All three types of endothelins can be released during brain insults, either from damaged endothelium or from astroglia. Functional endothelin receptors of ET_B type have been shown in cultured microglial cells, where they control $InsP_3$-induced Ca^{2+} release from the ER. Astrocytes express ET_A and ET_B receptors; activation of astroglial receptors decreases expression of gap junctions and therefore inhibits coupling in the astroglial networks.

5.3.7 Platelet-activating factor receptors

Platelet-activating factor (PAF) is a potent biological mediator; it activates platelets and has various effects on other tissues, including CNS, where it is involved in regulation of neuronal plasticity, inflammation, apoptosis, etc. The PAF receptors are found in microglia, where their activation induces a robust $[Ca^{2+}]_i$ elevation, originating from both Ca^{2+} release from the ER and Ca^{2+} influx. PAF receptors have also been identified in cultured astrocytes; activation of astroglial PAF receptors may induce the release of prostaglandins and may also mediate cell death.

5.3.8 Thrombin receptors

Thrombin is a serine-protease, which is involved in blood coagulation; besides, thrombin triggers various responses in both peripheral tissues and neural cells. The thrombin receptors, which belong to a protease-activated receptor family, have been identified in microglial cells, where they triggered $InsP_3$-induced Ca^{2+} release and inhibited store-operated Ca^{2+} entry. Similar receptors are present in astrocytes, where they may be implicated in initiation of reactive gliosis.

5.4 Glial syncytium – gap junctions

Macroglial cells in the brain are physically connected, forming a functional cellular syncytium. This represents a fundamental difference between neuronal and glial networking. For the vast majority of neurones, networking is provided by synaptic contacts. The latter preclude physical continuity of the neuronal network, while providing for functional inter-neuronal signal propagation. In contrast, glial networks are supported by direct intercellular contacts, generally known as *gap junctions*.

The *gap junctions* are, in fact, present in many types of mammalian cells, where they are responsible for metabolic (e.g. in liver) and electrical (e.g. in the heart) coupling. At the ultrastructural level (seen by electron microscopy, EM, and freeze fracture EM), gap junctions appear as specialized areas where two apposing membranes of adjacent cells come very close together, so that the intercellular cleft is reduced to a width of about 2–2.5 nm. Within these areas, each gap junction is made up of many hundreds of intercellular channels comprised of specialized proteins known as *connexons*; these form an intercellular channel which is in essence a large aqueous pore connecting the cytoplasm of both adjacent cells (Figure 5.7). Each intercellular channel is thus composed of two precisely aligned connexons (also known as hemichannels), one in each of the cell membranes of the two adjacent coupled cells.

On a molecular level, each connexon is composed of six symmetrical subunits, named *connexins*; hence, a functional intercellular channel comprises two connexons made up of twelve connexins. The connexins are many, and about 20 subtypes have been identified in mammalian tissues. These subtypes differ in

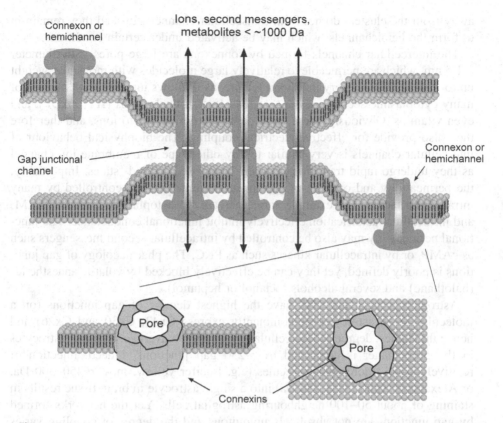

Figure 5.7 Structure of gap junctions – these are intercellular channels between two closely apposed cellular membranes, with the gap between cells ~2–3 nm wide. The intercellular channels are formed by two apposed hemichannels or connexons. Each connexon, in turn, is composed from six subunits known as connexins (see the text for further explanation). The gap junction channels permit intercellular movement of solutes with a m.w. up to 1000 Da, such as ions, second messengers and metabolites

molecular weight (which varies between 26 kDa and 62 kDa), which is used in connexin nomenclature, e.g. Cx43 and Cx32 are the most abundant connexins in astrocytes and oligodendrocytes, respectively. Each connexin has four transmembrane domains, which form the channel pore and gating mechanism.

The connexons may be formed from identical connexins (and then they are called *homomeric*), or several different connexins (*heteromeric*). Similarly, connexons in adjacent cells can be identical (making a *homotypic* gap junctional channel) or different (and then the channel is called *heterotypic*).

To produce a functional gap junction, several tens to hundreds of connexons must form a cluster; these clusters may connect similar cells (e.g. astrocyte to astrocyte) making a *homocellular gap junction*, or different cells (e.g. astrocyte and oligodendrocyte) forming a *heterocellular gap junction*. The connexons positioned away from the clusters do not form transcellular channels; instead they remain in to form the hemichannels, which may be activated under certain conditions.

The intercellular channels formed by connexons are large pores with diameter ~1.5 nm, which are permeable to relatively large molecules with molecular weight up to 1 kDa. This is a very important feature, as it allows intercellular diffusion of many cytoplasmic second messengers (e.g. $InsP_3$), nucleotides (ATP, ADP), and even vitamins. Obviously, these large pores are permeable to ions, and therefore they also provide for effective electrical coupling. The biophysical behaviour of intercellular channels is very similar to any other type of membrane ion channel as they undergo rapid transition between 'open' and 'closed' states. Importantly, the permeability and opening of gap junctional channels are controlled by many intracellular factors. For example, large increases in cytoplasmic Ca^{2+} (>10 μM) and intracellular acidification effectively inhibit junctional conductance. The junctional permeability may also be controlled by intracellular second messengers such as cAMP, or by intracellular kinases such as PKC. The pharmacology of gap junctions is poorly defined, yet they can be effectively blocked by volatile anaesthetics (halothane) and several alcohols (octanol or heptanol).

Astroglial cells in the CNS have the highest density of gap junctions (on a molecular level, astrocytes predominantly express Cx43, Cx30 and Cx26) and hence the highest degree of intercellular coupling. On average, a pair of astrocytes in the grey matter is connected by ~230 gap junctions. Indeed, injection of relatively small fluorescent molecules (e.g. Lucifer yellow, m.w. ~450–500 Da, or Alexa dyes with m.w. ~450 Da) into a single astrocyte in brain tissue results in staining of about 50–100 neighbouring astroglial cells. Yet the networks formed by gap junctions are not absolutely ubiquitous and the degree of coupling varies considerably between different brain regions. For example, almost all cortical astrocytes are integrated into the syncytium, whereas in the optic nerve the degree of coupling reaches ~80 per cent and in hippocampus it is much lower, being around ~50 per cent.

Oligodendrocytes also express several subtypes of connexins (Cx29, Cx32, Cx45, Cx47) and form both homocellular gap junctions with adjacent oligodendrocytes and heterocellular gap junctions with astroglial cells. Coupling between oligodendrocytes is much weaker compared to astrocytes, and usually every oligodendrocyte is coupled with two to four of its neighbours. The degree of this coupling is very different between various brain regions and also between species. Very often oligodendrocytes form gap junctions with astrocytes, the latter providing a general integrating media, which forms a 'panglial syncytium' within the brain. This integration also extends to ependymal cells, as the latter form gap junctions with astrocytes and also with other ependymocytes (Figure 5.8). Astrocytes may occasionally form gap junctional contacts with neurones, especially at early developmental stages.

Resting microglia do not contact each other and are not coupled to each other or to other glia (although activated microglia can express Cx43 *in vitro*). Similarly, NG2-glia are not functionally coupled to each other or to other glia; it is not known

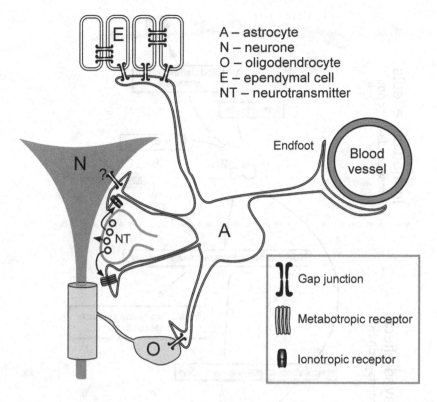

A – astrocyte
N – neurone
O – oligodendrocyte
E – ependymal cell
NT – neurotransmitter

Endfoot

Blood vessel

Gap junction

Metabotropic receptor

Ionotropic receptor

Figure 5.8 Gap junctions are instrumental in forming a panglial syncytium in the CNS. Astrocytes are considered to form a glial syncytium via extensive gap junctional communication. The scheme shows astrocytes forming gap junction contacts with each other and with oligodendrocytes, ependymal cells, and maybe even with some neurones. In addition, astrocytes receive chemical signals from synapses, and completely ensheath blood vessels with their perivascular endfeet. In this way, astrocytes integrate the brain into a functional syncytium

whether they express connexins. The lack of coupling in microglia and NG2-glia enables them to act individually in isolation from the glial syncytium, which may be particularly important at sites of brain injury.

Schwann cells express Cx32 and Cx46. Immature Schwann cells express Cx46 during development and following injury and are coupled to one another, whereas myelinating Schwann cells express Cx32, which connect paranodal loops of the myelin sheaths, where they are involved in ion and water movement.

5.5 Glial calcium signalling

Calcium ions are the most versatile and universal intracellular messengers discovered so far. They are involved in the regulation of almost all known cellular functions and reactions. The exceptions are few, the most notable probably being

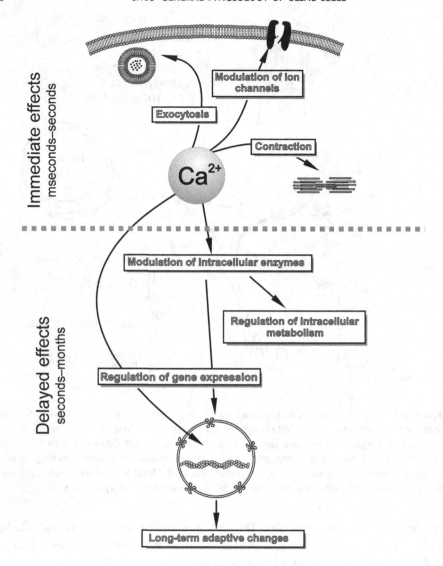

Figure 5.9 Versatility and ubiquity of calcium signalling. Calcium signals occur within different spatial and temporal domains controlling a wide variety of physiological reactions, ranging from immediate (exocytosis, modulation of ion channels, muscle contraction), to delayed (memory and long-term adaptive processes; see the text for further explanation). (From Toescu EC, Verkhratsky A (1998) Principles of calcium signalling. In: *Integrative Aspects of Calcium Signalling*, Verkhratsky A Toescu EC, Eds, Plenum Press, p. 2–22)

the propagation of nerve action potentials, which depends on Na^+ and K^+ channels that are not acutely Ca^{2+}-regulated. The most important properties of Ca^{2+} signalling are the promiscuity with respect to its effector systems and its auto-regulation. Indeed, Ca^{2+} regulates a truly remarkable variety of intracellular processes, within extremely different temporal domains, from microseconds (e.g. exocytosis) to months or even years (e.g. memory processes – see Figure 5.9). Physiological effects of Ca^{2+} ions are produced by intracellular Ca^{2+} sensors, represented by enzymes, which, upon Ca^{2+} binding, change their activity. These enzymes have different affinity and therefore sensitivity to Ca^{2+} ions (e.g. Ca^{2+} sensors in the cytosol are regulated by Ca^{2+} in concentrations of hundreds of nM, whereas Ca^{2+}-dependent enzymes in the endoplasmic reticulum are sensitive to Ca^{2+} concentrations in the range of 100–1000 μM). Furthermore the intracellular Ca^{2+} sensors are localized in different parts of the cell, and therefore local Ca^{2+} gradients may specifically regulate particular sets of Ca^{2+}-dependent processes. These peculiarities of intracellular Ca^{2+} effector systems allow for amplitude and space encoding of Ca^{2+} signals and solve the problem of specificity of such an intrinsically promiscuous system.

The actual molecular systems responsible for controlling intracellular Ca^{2+} homeostasis and producing Ca^{2+} signalling events are limited to several protein families represented by *Ca^{2+} channels* and *Ca^{2+} transporters*. These systems are very much conserved and ubiquitously expressed within the cellular kingdom. Most importantly, all these systems are regulated by Ca^{2+} itself, thus making a very robust, albeit versatile and adaptable piece of molecular machinery.

5.5.1 Cellular Ca^{2+} regulation

The free intracellular Ca^{2+} represents only a small ($\sim$0.001 per cent) fraction of total cellular calcium. Within the cells free Ca^{2+} is very unevenly distributed between intracellular compartments. Cytosolic free Ca^{2+} concentration ($[Ca^{2+}]_i$) is very low, being in the range of 50–100 nM. Calcium concentration within the ER is much higher, varying between 0.2 and 1.0 mM, and being therefore similar to extracellular Ca^{2+} concentration, which lies around 1.5–2.0 mM (Figure 5.10). As a result of these concentration differences an extremely large electrochemical driving force keeps the cytosol under continuous 'Ca^{2+} pressure', as Ca^{2+} ions try to diffuse from the high concentration regions to the compartment with low free Ca^{2+}.

These distinct compartments, however, are separated by biological membranes (the plasma membrane and endomembrane separate the cytosol from the extra-cellular and ER compartments, respectively). Movement of Ca^{2+} between the compartments therefore requires specific systems, represented by several super-families of transmembrane Ca^{2+}-permeable channels, ATP-driven Ca^{2+} pumps and electrochemically-driven Ca^{2+} exchangers. The Ca^{2+} fluxes resulting from the activity of these systems may either deliver or remove Ca^{2+} from the cytoplasm (Figure 5.11).

Major routes for plasmalemmal Ca^{2+} entry are provided by *voltage-gated, ligand-gated and nonspecific channels* (Figure 5.11), which have distinct activation

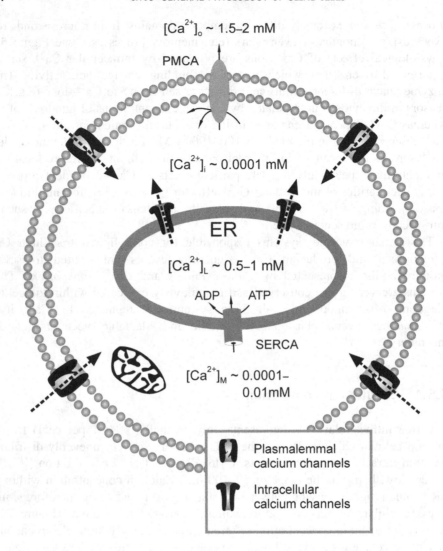

Figure 5.10 Cellular calcium gradients. Concentration of free calcium differs considerably between the cytosol and extracellular solution and cytosol and intracellular organelles. The $[Ca^{2+}]_i$ in the cytosol is ~20 000 times lower than in the extracellular milieu and ~10 000 times lower than within the lumen of endoplasmic reticulum, which creates huge gradients aimed at the cytoplasm and underlying rapid generation of cytosolic calcium signals. See Figure 5.11 for abbreviations

mechanisms and differ in their Ca^{2+} permeability. Plasmalemmal voltage-gated Ca^{2+} channels are the most selective for Ca^{2+} ions, whereas other channels allow the passage of Ca^{2+} and other cations; for example AMPA type glutamate receptors are principally ligand-gated Na^+/K^+ channels, but also display permeability to Ca^{2+}. Due to a very steep concentration gradient for Ca^{2+} between the

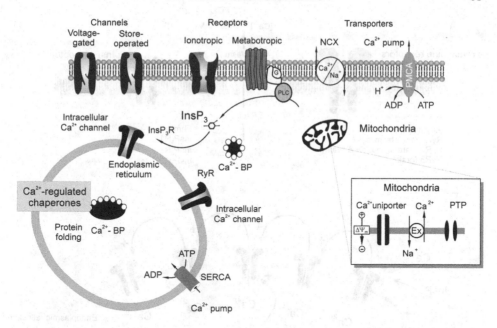

Figure 5.11 Molecular cascades of cellular calcium homeostasis. Calcium homeostasis and the calcium signalling system results from concerted interaction of Ca^{2+} channels (which include plasmalemmal ion channels, ionotropic receptors and intracellular Ca^{2+} channels), Ca^{2+} transporters (Ca^{2+} pumps and Na^+/Ca^{2+} exchanger, NCX) and cellular Ca^{2+} buffers. Ca^{2+} channels provide pathways for Ca^{2+} entry into the cytosol, whereas Ca^{2+} transporters accomplish Ca^{2+} translocation against concentration gradients either back to the extracellular space or into the lumen of the ER. Mitochondria also act as dynamic Ca^{2+} buffers; mitochondrial Ca^{2+} accumulation occurs through the Ca^{2+} uniporter (highly selective Ca^{2+} channel) down the electro-chemical gradient (intra-mitochondrial potential is −200 mV relative to the cytosol); whereas Ca^{2+} can be released from mitochondria via NCX (Na^+–Ca^{2+} exchanger), or (especially in pathological conditions) via permeability transition pore (PTP). See the text for further details.

Abbreviations: NCX – Na^+/Ca^{2+} exchanger; PMCA – Plasmalemmal Calcium ATP-ase; Ca^{2+}–BP – Ca^{2+} binding proteins; $InsP_3R$ – Inositol-1,4,5-trisphosphate Receptor/Inositol-1,4,5-trisphosphate-gated Ca^{2+} channel; RyR – Ryanodine Receptors/Ca^{2+}-gated Ca^{2+} channel; SERCA – Sarco(Endo)plasmic Reticulum Calcium ATPase. Intra-ER Ca^{2+} binding proteins also act as Ca^{2+} dependent chaperones, which are enzymes controlling protein folding into the tertiary structure

extracellular space and the cytosol, opening of even a small number of plasmalemmal Ca^{2+} channels results in a relatively large Ca^{2+} influx, which may rapidly change cytosolic free Ca^{2+}. The second important source of cytosolic Ca^{2+} ions is associated with release from the ER, which serves as an intracellular Ca^{2+} store; in fact the ER Ca^{2+} store acts as the main source for cytoplasmic Ca^{2+} signals in nonexcitable cells. From the ER, Ca^{2+} is delivered to the cytosol via two classes of ligand-gated Ca^{2+} channels residing in the endomembrane, namely *ryanodine receptors (RyR)* and *InsP$_3$ receptors (InsP$_3$R)* (Figure 5.12).

RyR are activated by cytosolic Ca^{2+} ions, and therefore act as an amplifier of Ca^{2+} signals; these Ca^{2+} channels are generally known as RyR because they are

A

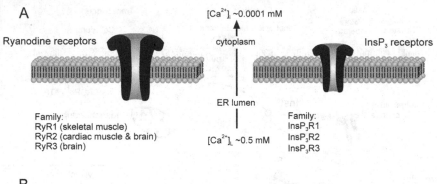

Ryanodine receptors

$[Ca^{2+}]_i$ ~0.0001 mM

cytoplasm

InsP$_3$ receptors

ER lumen

Family:
RyR1 (skeletal muscle)
RyR2 (cardiac muscle & brain)
RyR3 (brain)

$[Ca^{2+}]_L$ ~0.5 mM

Family:
InsP$_3$R1
InsP$_3$R2
InsP$_3$R3

B

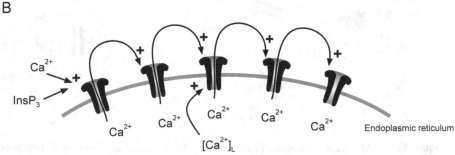

Ca^{2+}

InsP$_3$

Ca^{2+}

Ca^{2+}

Ca^{2+}

Ca^{2+}

Ca^{2+}

Ca^{2+}

$[Ca^{2+}]_L$

Endoplasmic reticulum

Figure 5.12 Mechanisms of calcium release from the endoplasmic reticulum:
A. Intracellular Ca^{2+} release channels are represented by two families of Ca^{2+}-gated Ca^{2+} channels, or Ryanodine receptors (RyRs), and InsP$_3$-gated Ca^{2+} channels, or InsP$_3$ receptors.
B. Mechanism of propagating intracellular Ca^{2+} waves is determined by the Ca^{2+} sensitivity of both RyRs and InsP$_3$Rs; local increases in $[Ca^{2+}]_i$ activate neighbouring channels and produce a propagating wave of excitation of ER-resident Ca^{2+} release channels

selectively activated (at low concentrations, < 1 μM) or inhibited (at 50–100 μM) by the plant alkaloid ryanodine. The activation of RyR is also regulated by the naturally occurring intracellular second messenger cyclic ADP ribose. There are three types of RyRs, the RyR1 (or 'skeletal muscle' type), the RyR2 (or 'cardiac muscle' type) and the RyR3 (or 'brain' type); although their names are misleading, as they are not only expressed in these tissues; moreover RyR3 expression in the CNS is actually relatively minor. RyR1 can establish direct contacts with plasmalemmal voltage-gated Ca^{2+} channels, and the opening of the latter upon depolarization will also open RyR1 and trigger *depolarization-induced Ca^{2+} release* (which does not require Ca^{2+} entry and Ca^{2+} interactions with the ER channel). RyR2 and RyR3 can be activated only by an increase in cytosolic $[Ca^{2+}]_i$, thus producing a *calcium-induced Ca^{2+} release*.

InsP$_3$R   Ca^{2+} channels are activated by the intracellular second messenger InsP$_3$, which triggers *InsP$_3$-induced Ca^{2+} release*. Importantly, InsP$_3$Rs are also regulated by cytosolic free Ca^{2+}, so that elevation of the latter increases the sensitivity of the receptors to InsP$_3$; high (>1 μM) [Ca^{2+}]$_i$ inhibits type 1 InsP$_3$R, but not type 2 and 3.

Elementary Ca^{2+} release events associated with opening of a single RyR or InsP$_3$R are respectively known as Ca^{2+} *sparks* or *puffs*; summation of the local events produce a global increase in [Ca^{2+}]$_i$. All in all, release of Ca^{2+} from several ER channels activates neighbouring RyRs and InsP$_3$Rs, thereby creating a propagating wave of ER excitation; by this means Ca^{2+} signals are able to travel intracellularly for long distances within polarized cells (Figure 5.12 B).

Importantly, the ER and plasmalemma are functionally linked through a specific class of plasmalemmal channels known as '*store-operated Ca^{2+} channels*' (SOCCs; this pathway is also known as a 'capacitative' Ca^{2+} entry). The latter provide for additional Ca^{2+} influx in conditions when the ER is depleted from Ca^{2+}; this additional influx helps to replenish the ER Ca^{2+} stores.

Upon entering the cytoplasm, many Ca^{2+} ions are immediately bound by *Ca^{2+}-binding proteins* (e.g. calbindin 28K), which determine the Ca^{2+}-buffering capacity of the cytoplasm; Ca^{2+} ions that escape binding, and therefore stay free, generate an intracellular Ca^{2+} signalling event. The cytoplasmic buffering capacity of different cells varies substantially; for example in a cerebellar Purkinje neurone only 1 out of 4000 Ca^{2+} ions remain free; in hippocampal neurones this ratio equals 1:70–150.

Excess Ca^{2+} ions entering the cytoplasm during stimulation are removed by several plasmalemmal and intracellular transporters, which expel Ca^{2+} from the cytosol against a concentration gradient and prevent the system from overloading. Plasmalemmal Ca^{2+} extrusion is achieved by Ca^{2+} pumps (*PMCA, plasmalemmal Ca^{2+} ATPase*), which use the energy of ATP hydrolysis to transport Ca^{2+}, and by *sodium–calcium exchanger* (*NCX*), which uses the electrochemical gradient of Na$^+$ ions as the driving force for Ca^{2+} efflux (extrusion of every Ca^{2+} ion requires entry of 3–4 Na$^+$ ions into the cell, and is dependent on the Na$^+$ concentration gradient maintained by the activity of Na$^+$-K$^+$ pumps). A size-able amount of Ca^{2+} is also removed from the cytosol by active uptake into the lumen of the ER via the *SERCA pumps* (*Sarco(Endo)plasmic Reticulum Ca^{2+} ATPases*) residing in the endomembrane. The activity of SERCA pumps is strongly regulated by the free Ca^{2+} concentration within the ER, and depletion of the ER from Ca^{2+} ions significantly increases the capacity of the SERCA to pump Ca^{2+} ions.

All these extrusion systems are assisted by the mitochondria, which are endowed with a very selective Ca^{2+} channel known as the '*Ca^{2+} uniporter*'. As the mito-chondrial inner membrane is very electronegative compared to the cytosol (up to –200 mV), elevations of cytosolic Ca^{2+} above ~0.5 μM drive Ca^{2+} ions along the electrochemical gradient into the mitochondria. On entering mitochondria, Ca^{2+} ions activate ATP synthesis and provide a mechanism for coupling cell stimulation with energy production.

Finally, it should be noted that excessive stimulation of Ca^{2+} influx into the cytosol has a detrimental effect, being the main mechanism of so-called '*Ca^{2+}*

excitotoxicity'. The latter occurs during long-lasting excessive stimulation of Ca^{2+} entry, e.g. by pathological release of glutamate during brain ischaemia, or by failure of Ca^{2+} extrusion systems, usually through lack of energy. Long-lasting increases in $[Ca^{2+}]_i$ in turn stimulate various enzymatic pathways that initiate apoptotic or necrotic cell death.

5.5.2   Glial Ca^{2+} signalling – endoplasmic reticulum takes the leading role

Glial cells have all the components of Ca^{2+} homeostatic/signalling machinery discussed above. An important difference between glial cells and neurones, however, is the relative scarcity of voltage-gated Ca^{2+} channels in glial cells. The majority of mature astrocytes, oligodendrocytes and Schwann cells do not express voltage-gated Ca^{2+} channels. Nonetheless, voltage-gated Ca^{2+} currents are present in immature astroglial cells and oligodendrocyte precursors, and their expression is down-regulated during development. It is likely that voltage-gated Ca^{2+} channels are involved in growth and differentiation of glial cells.

Ca^{2+} entry pathways in mature glial cells are represented by several types of Ca^{2+} permeable ligand-gated channels (most notably by ionotropic glutamate and P2X purinoreceptors) and store-operated Ca^{2+} channels.

The main source for glial Ca^{2+} signalling is associated with the ER Ca^{2+} store. The intra-ER Ca^{2+} concentration in glial cells varies between 100–300 μM, thus being lower compared to neurones (where intra-ER free Ca^{2+} reaches 300–800 μM). All types of glial cells express numerous metabotropic receptors and their activation causes an increase in cytosolic concentration of $InsP_3$, which binds to the $InsP_3Rs$ and causes rapid Ca^{2+} release. It seems that $InsP_3$-induced Ca^{2+} release represents the leading mechanism of Ca^{2+} signalling in glia. Although both astrocytes and microglia express RyRs, they play a relatively minor (if any) role in shaping Ca^{2+} signals in these cells. The RyRs are more important in OPCs and immature oligodendrocytes, where they are directly coupled to voltage-gated Ca^{2+} channels located in the plasma membrane along processes. Thus, opening of voltage-gated Ca^{2+} channels activates RyRs and triggers depolarization-induced Ca^{2+} release, providing a potential mechanism by which axonal electrical activity may regulate oligodendroglial Ca^{2+} signals and process outgrowth.

The release of Ca^{2+} from intracellular stores lowers intra-ER Ca^{2+} concentration, which in turn triggers opening of SOCC, which are abundantly present in all types of glial cells. Although the molecular nature of these channels and details of their activation mechanism are unknown, they are functionally very important, as their activation produces prolonged Ca^{2+} signals, which may significantly outlast the duration of stimulation.

The interplay between Ca^{2+} release, Ca^{2+} reuptake into the ER and SOCC-related Ca^{2+} entry determines the shape of the resulting Ca^{2+} signal, which may vary from a rapid and transient peak-like response, through $[Ca^{2+}]_i$ elevations lasting up to hundreds of seconds with a clear plateau, to multiple transient Ca^{2+} oscillations. These kinetically different $[Ca^{2+}]_i$ changes underlie the temporal coding of the Ca^{2+} signal, whereas $[Ca^{2+}]_i$ oscillations are responsible for frequency coding of the Ca^{2+} signal.

5.5.3 Propagating calcium waves as a substrate of glial excitability

In physiological conditions, glia are stimulated by relatively brief and local exposures to neurotransmitters. This local stimulation produces similarly localized events of Ca^{2+} release through $InsP_3R$; yet these highly localized events (which in essence are a summation of several puffs) may give rise to a propagating signal that will swamp the whole cell. Importantly in glial cells, particularly in astrocytes, propagation of these Ca^{2+} waves is not limited by cellular borders; instead they cross the intercellular boundaries and spread over a relatively long distance through the astrocytic syncytium.

Intracellular propagation of Ca^{2+} signals is determined by a special property of the ER membrane, which, similar to the plasmalemma of excitable cells, is able to convert a local supra-threshold response into a propagating wave of excitation. The Ca^{2+} sensitivity of the RyRs and $InsP_3Rs$ is what makes the ER membrane an excitable medium. A focal Ca^{2+} release induced by a localized elevation of $InsP_3$ recruits neighbouring channels, which not only amplifies the initial Ca^{2+} release event, but also creates a propagating wave of Ca^{2+} release along the ER membrane. This simple mechanism underlies the propagation of Ca^{2+} signals in almost any type of nonexcitable cell. It is important to remember that the Ca^{2+} wave is not a propagating wave of Ca^{2+} ions, because the movement of Ca^{2+} ions is severely restricted by cytoplasmic Ca^{2+} buffering. Instead, the Ca^{2+}wave results from a propagating wave of elementary Ca^{2+} release events through the endomembrane.

Intercellular propagation of Ca^{2+} signals is primarily a function of astrocytes, and involves several mechanisms, including: (1) direct intercellular diffusion of $InsP_3$ via gap junctions; (2) regenerative release of a diffusible extracellular messenger (e.g. ATP) triggering metabotropic receptor-mediated Ca^{2+} release in neighbouring cells; (3) diffusion of an extracellular messenger after release from a single cell (which may be important in microglia as well as astrocytes); and (4) any combination of the above (see schemes on Figure 5.13). Astroglial networks in different areas of the brain can have distinct mechanisms of intercellular Ca^{2+} wave propagation. For example, genetic deletion of Cx43, which forms gap junctions between brain astrocytes (see Chapter 5.4), results in the complete disappearance of astroglial Ca^{2+} waves in the neocortex, but not in the corpus callosum or hippocampus, where Ca^{2+} wave propagation relies primarily on ATP release. Furthermore, intercellular Ca^{2+} waves can be propagated outside

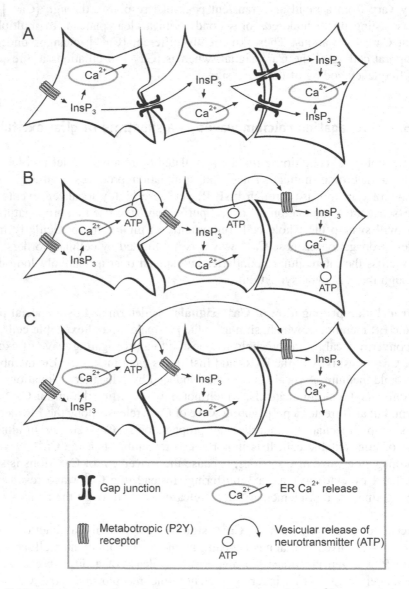

Figure 5.13 Mechanisms of generation of propagating intercellular Ca^{2+} waves. Propagation of inter-glial Ca^{2+} waves can be supported by several distinct mechanisms, which can operate separately or in combination:

A. Ca^{2+} waves can be maintained by diffusion of $InsP_3$ through the gap junction and secondary initiation of $InsP_3$-induced Ca^{2+} release;

B. Ca^{2+} waves can be maintained by regenerative Ca^{2+}-dependent release of 'gliotransmitters' (see Figure 5.14) acting on neighbouring cells through extracellular diffusion;

C. Ca^{2+} waves can result from a focal release of 'gliotransmitter', which then diffuses over a long distance.

of the astroglial syncytium by the release of extracellular messengers to act on neighbouring neurones, oligodendrocytes and microglia.

Intercellular Ca^{2+} waves may travel for 300–400 μm at a velocity of ~15–20 μm/s, and provide astrocytes with the means for long-distance communication. Thus, astrocytes are 'excitable', but signal propagation is fundamentally different from that in neurones. In neurones, the substrate for excitability is the plasma membrane, which generates a rapidly (milliseconds) propagating wave of openings/closures of Na^+/K^+ channels (propagating action potential). In contrast, the substrate for excitability in astrocytes is the intracellular ER membrane, which generates a much slower (seconds to minutes) propagating wave of openings/closures of Ca^{2+} channels.

5.6 Neurotransmitter release from astroglial cells

Neurotransmitters such as glutamate, ATP, GABA etc. are the material substrates of synaptic transmission, and their regulated release in the CNS was, for many years, believed to be a sole prerogative of neurones and neuro-endocrine cells. Experimental investigations of glial cells performed over the last 15 years, however, have clearly demonstrated that at least some neurotransmitters can be released from astroglial cells (Table 5.3). Thus, chemical transmission is the universal mechanism for communication between both neurones and astrocytes (it has not yet been established that oligodendrocytes, microglia or NG2-glia release neurotransmitters, but they clearly respond to neurotransmitters released by

Table 5.3 'Glio' transmitters

Neurotransmitter	Mechanism of release	Function
Glutamate	Vesicular, hemichannels, $P2X_7$ receptors	Activation of neuronal glutamate receptors
Aspartate	Hemichannels	Activation of neuronal glutamate receptors
ATP	Vesicular, hemichannels	Activation of neuronal and glial purinoreceptors; initiation of propagating calcium waves though glial syncytium
D-serine	Transporter (?); vesicular (?)	Activation of neuronal NMDA receptors
Homocysteine	??	Activation of neuronal NMDA receptors
Taurine	Volume-activated chloride channels	Activation of glycine receptors in supraoptic nuclei and circumventricular organ

neurones and astrocytes). Neurotransmitters can be released from astrocytes via several pathways, generally classified as nonvesicular and vesicular, the difference being determined by whether transmitter was accumulated into specialized vesicles before release, or, alternatively, was released directly from the cytosol.

5.6.1 Nonvesicular release of neurotransmitter from astrocytes

Several types of neurotransmitters, including glutamate, ATP and aspartate, can be released from astrocytes through plasmalemmal routes, namely via reversed activity of neurotransmitter transporters or via plasmalemmal channels (Figure 5.14).

Reversed activity of transporters can result in glutamate release from astrocytes (and maybe also from oligodendrocytes); this can happen in conditions of increased intracellular concentrations of Na^+ or glutamate, combined with cell depolarization caused by an increased extracellular concentration of K^+. These conditions are clearly pathological and may occur in ischaemia and upon various insults to CNS, which are accompanied by neuronal damage and massive release of glutamate and

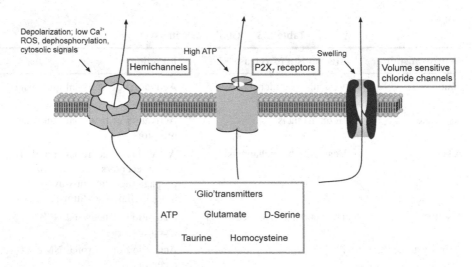

Figure 5.14 Mechanisms of nonvesicular 'gliotransmitter' release from astrocytes. Nonvesicular release of gliotransmitters can occur through volume-sensitive chloride channels, through hemichannels or through P2X$_7$ receptors; all these channels can allow passage of relatively large molecules with m.w. up to 1 kDa

K^+ into the extracellular space. Glutamate in turn is accumulated by astrocytes together with Na^+.

Volume-activated anion channels provide a route for the release of glutamate and other negatively charged amino acids, such as taurine. These volume-activated anion channels are opened upon hypo-osmotic shock, i.e. by a decrease in extracellular osmotic pressure, which in turn leads to rapid swelling of astroglial cells. This type of release is physiologically important in the supraoptic nerve of the hypothalamus, which is the primary centre of body osmoregulation. Minor changes (several percentages) of extracellular osmotic pressure stimulate (hypo-osmotic conditions) or inhibit (hyper-osmotic conditions) taurine release from hypophysal glial cells (pituicytes); taurine in turn interacts with glycine receptors present in the terminals of vasopressin/oxytocin neurones, thereby regulating secretion of these two neuro-hormones, which are important in regulation of overall body osmotic homeostasis.

Hemichannels that do not form gap junctions (see Chapter 5.4) provide a further route for glutamate, aspartate and ATP release from astroglial cells. Release of neurotransmitters through this pathway may be regulated, for example, by physiological changes in intra- or extracellular Ca^{2+} concentration.

P2X$_7$ purinoreceptors are large enough to be permeable to amino acid molecules (see Chapter 5.3.2) and may also constitute a pathway by which neurotransmitters can be released from astrocytes, although it must be noted that $P2X_7$ receptors are most likely activated under pathological conditions when extracellular ATP rises above $\sim$1 mM.

5.6.2 Vesicular release of neurotransmitter from glial cells

Vesicular release, also known as exocytosis, is the main pathway for regulated secretion of neurochemicals by neurones. Exocytosis underlies the very rapid Ca^{2+}-dependent release of neurotransmitter in neuronal synapses as well as the much slower (also Ca^{2+}-dependent) process of secretion of various neuromodulators and neuro-hormones. An important feature of the exocytotic mechanism is that it is activated by local increases in intracellular Ca^{2+} concentration; the latter being produced either by plasmalemmal Ca^{2+} entry or by receptor-stimulated Ca^{2+} release from intracellular stores. Whatever the trigger for Ca^{2+} elevation, the resulting local Ca^{2+} signals represent the mechanism by which neurotransmitter release is coupled to stimulation, which underlies the coordinated activity of neural cells.

   In all cases, elevation of cytosolic Ca^{2+} is an essential triggering event, but neurosecretion then depends on several processes (Figure 5.15). The whole cycle

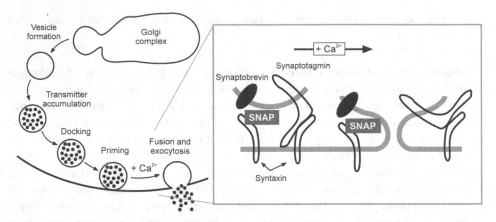

Figure 5.15 General mechanisms of exocytosis. The exocytotic cycle proceeds through several functionally distinct steps. First, the vesicles are formed in, and separated from, the Golgi complex. Subsequently vesicles accumulate transmitter, and are docked to the cellular membrane and primed for release. The act of exocytosis is triggered by local $[Ca^{2+}]_i$ microdomains (where Ca^{2+} concentration may rise up to $10–100\,\mu M$). Following exocytosis the excessive membranes are internalized via the endocytotic process and are transported back to the Golgi complex. The exocytotic process is controlled by several vesicular and plasmalemmal proteins, the most important of which are represented by syntaxin, synaptobrevin and synaptotagmin. Generation of local Ca^{2+} microdomains triggers conformational changes in exocytotic proteins, which results in vesicle fusion with the plasmalemma and release of vesicular contents

begins at the level of Golgi apparatus, where the vesicles containing the neuro-chemicals are produced and matured. Then, the vesicles are transported to the site of release, a process known as targeting. Consequently, targeted vesicles are prepared for exocytosis by docking and priming, after which local Ca^{2+} elevations trigger vesicle fusion and release of secretory material. To repeat the cycle, the vesicles are retrieved from the plasmalemma, after which they return to the ER and Golgi complex.

The fusion of vesicles is controlled by several specialized proteins, located in the vesicle membrane and in the plasmalemma (Figure 5.15). The vesicle contains the actual Ca^{2+}-sensor, synaptotagmin I, and synaptobrevin II (or vesicle-associated membrane protein 2, VAMP2); whereas the plasmalemmal counterparts are represented by syntaxin and the protein SNAP25 (synaptosome-associated protein of m.w. 25 kDa). The latter three proteins form a core of the fusion mechanism and are summarily known as SNARE proteins ('soluble N-ethylmaleimide-sensitive factor (NSF)-associated protein receptors'). When the Ca^{2+} concentration in the vicinity of the primed and docked vesicle is increased, the synaptotagmin is activated, which in turn stimulates the formation of the complex between synaptobrevin II from the vesicular side and syntaxin and SNAP25 from the plasma membrane side, leading to the fusion of the vesicle with the cellular membrane (Figure 5.15). Of course, this description is very much simplified and in reality many other proteins assist and fine-tune the process, yet the described core events remain obligatory for every neurosecretory event known so far.

It is now evident that astrocytes possess all the major proteins involved in exocytosis; expression of all three members of the SNARE family as well as synaptotagmin I and several auxiliary exocytotic proteins (e.g. sectetogranin, synapsin I or Rab3) has been confirmed in numerous astroglial preparations. Furthermore, astrocytes have intracellular structures similar to synaptic microvesicles, which are endowed with vesicle-specific proteins (synaptobrevin) and have a particularly high concentration of glutamate. Astrocytes also contain vesicular glutamate transporters (VGLUT), which accumulate glutamate within vesicles. Sometimes, these astroglial glutamate-containing vesicles are gathered in astroglial processes, although nothing similar to a presynaptic pool of vesicles characteristic for neuronal terminals has ever been observed. NG2-glia have also been shown to form synapse-like connections with neurones, but it is not known whether they have the mechanisms for vesicular release of neurotransmitter.

Most importantly, astroglial release of glutamate in response to raised intracellular Ca^{2+} has been demonstrated directly. This glutamate release is stimulated by

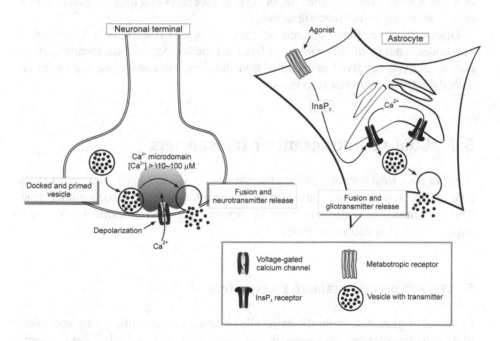

Figure 5.16 Neuronal and glial exocytosis: the source of Ca^{2+}. The fundamental difference between transmitter release from neuronal presynaptic terminals and from glial cells lies in the source of the Ca^{2+} trigger. In neurones, Ca^{2+} enters the presynaptic terminal via activation of voltage-gated plasmalemmal channels; this ensures very rapid $[Ca^{2+}]_i$ rise and fast exocytosis. In glial cells, Ca^{2+} comes from the intracellular stores, which results in a slower but more sustained $[Ca^{2+}]_i$ increase and hence slower but more sustained release of 'gliotransmitters'

activation of astroglial metabotropic receptors, e.g. P2Y purinoreceptors, mGluRs, bradykinin, and BDNF (Trk B) receptors, and is invariably sensitive to intracellular Ca^{2+} elevation, as chelation of intracellular Ca^{2+} with membrane-permeable Ca^{2+}-binding agents (e.g. BAPTA/AM) effectively inhibits the release.

Vesicular glutamate release from astrocytes is fundamentally different from that in neurones in respect to the source of trigger Ca^{2+}: in astrocytes, Ca^{2+} comes almost exclusively from the intracellular stores, whereas neuronal exocytosis is governed predominantly by Ca^{2+} entry through plasmalemmal channels (Figure 5.16). As a consequence, vesicular release of neurotransmitter from astroglial cells develops considerably slower compared to neurones. Another important peculiarity of glial vesicular release is associated with a specific type of exocytosis found in hippocampal astrocytes: these cells may exhibit a so-called 'kiss-and-run' exocytosis, when the secretory vesicles open for a very short period of time ($\sim$2 ms) and do not completely empty their contents.

Astroglial cells may also utilize vesicular exocytosis to secrete another neurotransmitter, D-serine. D-serine is synthesized by astrocytes from L-serine using the enzyme serine racemase, and can be regarded as a specific glial neurotransmitter. D-serine activates the 'glycine' site of NMDA receptors and may play an important role in astrocyte-to-neurone signalling.

Discovery of regulated NT release from astrocytes is extremely important for our understanding of mechanisms of brain functioning, as this means that glia may be actively involved in chemical transmission, and can (as we shall see later) directly activate neuronal responses.

5.7 Glial neurotransmitter transporters

Another important part of cellular glial physiology is associated with their remarkable ability to accumulate various neurotransmitters from the extracellular space. This accumulation is accomplished by several specific transporters, abundantly expressed in glial cell membranes.

5.7.1 Astrocyte glutamate transporters

Removal of glutamate from the extracellular space is accomplished by specialized glutamate transporters expressed in both neurones and astroglial cells. Normal extracellular glutamate concentration varies between 2 and 5 μM, reaching higher levels only for very brief moments at the peak of synaptic transmission. Intracellular glutamate concentration, in contrast, is much larger, being in the range of 1 to 10 mM. Therefore, removal of glutamate from the extracellular space requires transportation against a substantial concentration gradient. To perform this 'uphill' translocation, glutamate transporters utilize the transmembrane electrochemical gradients of Na^+ and K^+. Transport of a single glutamate molecule requires influx of three Na^+ ions and efflux of one K^+ ion, down their concentration gradients; in addition glutamate brings one more H^+ ion into the cell (Figure 5.17). The net influx of cations manifests the electrogenic effect of glutamate transporters, which appears in a form of an inward current; the latter depolarizes the cell, further assisting the uptake of negatively charged glutamate.

There are five types of glutamate transporters in the human brain, classified as EAAT1 to EAAT5 (where EAAT stands for Excitatory Amino Acid Transporter), out of which EAAT1 and EAAT2 are expressed in astrocytes, and the remaining three types are expressed in various types of neurones. Analogues of EAAT1 and EAAT 2 expressed in rat brain are known as GLAST (glutamate/aspartate transporter) and GLT-1 (glutamate transporter-1), respectively. Functional properties of all transporters are similar, although they differ slightly in their binding affinities for glutamate.

Astroglial expression of glutamate transporters is tightly controlled by neighbouring neurones (or most likely by the continuous presence of glutamate released during neuronal synaptic transmission). Removal of glutamatergic transmission or loss of neurones causes a significant down-regulation of astroglial glutamate transporter expression.

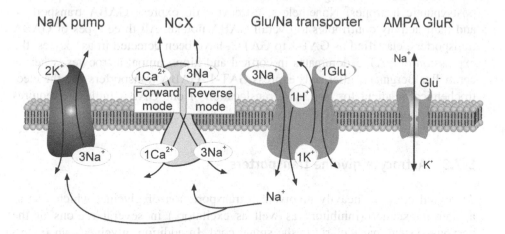

Figure 5.17 Ion fluxes generated by glutamate in glial cells and their relations to glutamate transport. Glutamate activates several molecular pathways and ion fluxes in astroglial cells. Glutamate activates ionotropic receptors and glutamate/Na^+ (Glu/Na) transporters, which results in a net Na^+ influx; the latter can increase intracellular Na^+ concentration from the resting level of $\sim$5 mM to 20–30 mM. This increase is counteracted by rapid reversal of the Na^+/Ca^{2+} exchanger (NCX), which expels excess Na^+ and provides Ca^{2+} entry, and a slower Na^+ extrusion through the Na^+/K^+ pump, which is energy-dependent. Maintenance of low intracellular Na^+ concentration is critically important for the performance of Na^+/glutamate transporter and glutamate uptake

The performance of glutamate transporters clearly depends on the transmembrane concentration gradients for Na^+ and K^+; an increase in intracellular Na^+ as well as an increase in extracellular K^+ hamper glutamate transport. In this sense, the uptake of glutamate is highly energy dependent, since maintaining the Na^+/K^+ concentration gradients requires ATP to fuel Na^+/K^+ pumps. On average, transportation of a single glutamate molecule requires ~1.5 molecules of ATP. Quite naturally, therefore, ATP depletion and disruption of Na^+/K^+ homeostasis, which inevitably accompany brain insults, inhibit astroglial glutamate uptake. Moreover, in certain conditions associated with severe energy deprivation and a significant increase in intracellular Na^+, the transporter can reverse and deliver glutamate into the extracellular space, thus further exacerbating excitotoxicity. Importantly, astrocytes express relatively high densities of sodium–calcium exchangers (NCX), which, upon an increase in cytosolic Na^+ concentration, are able to exchange Na^+ for Ca^{2+} (known as the reverse mode of NCX); this process may rapidly lower $[Na^+]_i$, therefore maintaining the operation of glutamate transporters (Figure 5.17).

5.7.2   Astrocyte GABA transporters

The role of astroglial cells in GABA uptake is not very prominent, as the majority of GABA released during neurotransmission is accumulated by both pre- and postsynaptic neurones. Nonetheless, astrocytes do express GABA transporters, and their activity contributes to overall GABA uptake. All three types of GABA transporters, classified as GAT-1 to GAT-3, have been detected in astrocytes; the expression of GAT-3 dominates in cortical and hippocampal astrocytes, whereas cerebellar Bergmann glial cells express GAT-1. GABA transporters use the electrochemical gradient for Na^+, and translocation of one GABA molecule requires a cotransportation of two Na^+ ions.

5.7.3   Astrocyte glycine transporters

Astroglial cells are heavily involved in transportation of glycine, which acts as a neurotransmitter (inhibitory as well as excitatory) in several regions of the nervous system, particularly in the spinal cord. In addition, glycine is an important neuromodulator acting on NMDA receptors throughout the brain. Glycine transporters present in neurones and astrocytes are functionally and structurally different. Astrocytes predominantly express Glycine transporter 1 (GlyT1), while neurones express GlyT2; both cotransport glycine with Na^+ and Cl^-, yet their stoichiometry is different. Glycine translocation by GlyT1 is coupled with cotransport of 2 Na^+ and 1 Cl^-, whereas GlyT2 requires cotransporting 3 Na^+ and 1 Cl^-. As a consequence, the reversal potential of glial GlyT1 is very close to the resting membrane potential, and therefore even a slight depolarization may promote the reversal of transporter and efflux of glycine into the extracellular space; this in turn can be important for modulating neuronal excitability. Neuronal GlyT2, in contrast is primarily involved with glycine clearance.

5.7.4 Other neurotransmitter transporters

Astroglial cells are able to transport various neurotransmitters and neuromodulators; the pattern and heterogeneity of neurotransmitter transporters expressed by astrocytes is dependent on the neurones they are associated with. Astrocytes can express transporters for monoamines (dopamine, norepinephrine and serotonin), yet the actual contribution of these uptake pathways in the regulation of brain monoamine levels remains undetermined. Astrocytes are reported to have a relatively high capacity for histamine uptake. In addition, certain astroglial cells express a Na^+/Cl^- dependent taurine transporting system, which is able to function in both forward (taurine uptake) and reverse (taurine release) modes. The reversal of the transporter requires cell depolarization (up to -50 mV) together with an increase in the intracellular Na^+ concentration above 40 mM; these conditions most likely may occur only during severe ischaemia. Functionally the taurine transporter (working in the forward mode) could be involved in taurine redistribution following a hypo-osmotic shock.

5.8 Glial cells produce and release neuropeptides

All types of glial cells produce and release neuropeptides (Table 5.4). The production of neuropeptides is highly region specific, and in many cases developmentally regulated. In particular, astroglial cells synthesize many types of opioid peptides such as enkephalins, which are involved in the regulation of cell proliferation and dendritic growth in the CNS. Similarly, opioids (proenkephalin and prodynorphin) are expressed in cells of the oligodendrocyte lineage, and may be involved in regulation of their development. Astrocytes in the cortex and cerebellum produce atrial natriuretic peptide, and are the main source of brain angiotensinogen; both peptides are involved in the regulation of brain water homeostasis. Some perivascular astrocytes also produce vasoactive intestinal polypeptide (VIP), which is involved in the regulation of the brain microcirculation. Neuropeptide Y (NPY) is heavily expressed by ensheathing cells of olfactory axons (olfactory ensheathing cells), where it is involved in promoting the growth of axons from olfactory epithelium to the olfactory bulb; similarly NPY is found in developing Schwann cells. The mechanisms of neuropeptide release from glial cells remain obscure. In some cases, it may involve exocytosis. This, for example, has been demonstrated for NPY, which is accumulated in vesicles present in olfactory ensheathing cells, and these vesicles can undergo Ca^{2+}-regulated exocytosis.

Table 5.4   Neuropeptides production and release in glial cells

Neuropeptide	Glial cell type	Function
Neuropeptide Y (NPY)	Ensheathing cells of the olfactory system Developing Schwann cells	Targeting axons to appropriate destination
Opioids (enkephalin, proenkephalins, dynorphin)	Astrocytes Oligodendrocyte precursors	Regulation of cell differentiation; control over dendritic growth
Angiotensinogen	Astrocytes in cortex and cerebellum	Part of brain renin–angiotensin system, regulation of water/ion homeostasis in the CNS
Atrial natriuretic peptide (ANP)	Astrocytes, Bergmann glia	Regulation of water/ion homeostasis in the CNS
Vasoactive intestinal peptide (VIP)	Astrocytes Pituicytes	Regulation of brain circulation (?)
Substance P	Astrocytes Microglia	Neuroinflammatory/damage mediator
Galanin	Oligodendrocyte precursors	Expression of galanin is controlled by thyroid hormone; galanin may be involved in regulation of growth and differentiation of neurones and oligodendrocytes
Carnosin	Astrocytes Tanycytes Ependyma Oligodendrocytes	??
Nociceptin	Astrocytes	??
Oxytocin and vasopressin	Pituicytes	??
Somatostatin	Astrocytes	??

5.9   Glial cell derived growth factors

Neurotrophic factors are polypeptides that regulate survival and differentiation of neural cells; a huge array of these neurotrophic factors are produced by glial cells. Particularly important are neurotrophins (the nerve growth factor, NGF; neurotrophins 3 and 4, NT-3, NT-4, and brain-derived neurotrophic factor, BDNF), which control a wide variety of CNS functions, from cell growth and differentiation, to synaptic transmission, regulation of ion channels expression and repair of neural circuits.

Glial cells produce and release growth factors in physiological conditions and upon neuronal damage. In the former case, growth factors derived from glia regulate various aspects of differentiation, growth and development of neural cells; whereas in the latter case, they help the processes responsible for regeneration and repair. In development, growth factors derived from glial cells regulate migration of neuronal precursors and immature neurones towards their final destiny, assist neuronal pathfinding, regulate appearance and remodelling of synaptic ensembles, and control ontogenetic nerve cell death. Astrocytes are the most prolific producers of growth factors; oligodendrocytes manufacture much less, but importantly they release netrin-1, which guides axonal pathfinding (and which is absent in astrocytes). Neuronal damage very much up-regulates production and release of growth factors especially from reactive astrocytes and activated microglial cells.

6

Neuronal–Glial Interactions

6.1 Close apposition of neurones and astroglia: the tripartite synapse

In the grey matter, astrocytes are closely associated with neuronal membranes and specifically with synaptic regions, so that in many cases astroglial membranes completely or partially enwrap presynaptic terminals as well as postsynaptic structures. In the hippocampus, for example, ~60 per cent of all axon–dendritic synapses are surrounded by astroglial membranes. These astrocyte–synapse contacts show peculiar specificity: astroglial membranes enwrap about 80 per cent of large perforated synapses (which are probably the most functionally active), whereas only about half of small (known as macular) synapses are covered by glial membranes. In the cerebellum, glial–synaptic relations are even more intimate, as nearly all of the synapses formed by parallel fibres on the dendrites of Purkinje neurone are covered by the membranes of Bergmann glial cells; each individual Bergmann cell enwraps between 2000 and 6000 synaptic contacts. The terminal strictures of astrocytes, which cover the synaptic regions, have a rather complex morphology: the Bergmann glial cells, for example, send specialized appendages, which cover several synapses and form a relatively independent compartment (Figure 6.1). This cover is quite intimate as the distance between glial membranes and synaptic structures in cerebellum and hippocampus is as close as 1 μm. The very intimate morphological apposition of astrocytes and synaptic structures allow the former to be exposed to the neurotransmitters released from the synaptic terminals. Functionally, the processes of astroglial cells are endowed with neurotransmitter receptors, and most importantly, the modalities of receptors expressed by astroglial membranes precisely match the neurotransmitters released at the synapses they cover. In this respect, astrocytes in fact have a complement of receptors very similar to that of their neuronal neighbour. In the cerebellum, for example, the Purkinje neurone/Bergmann glia pair receives several synaptic inputs, which use as neurotransmitters glutamate, ATP, noradrenalin, histamine and GABA; both neurone and glial cell express receptors specific for these substances (see Chapter 5). In the cortex, both pyramidal neurones and neighbouring astroglial

Glial Neurobiology: A Textbook   Alexei Verkhratsky and Arthur Butt
© 2007 John Wiley & Sons, Ltd   ISBN 978-0-470-01564-3 (HB); 978-0-470-51740-6 (PB)

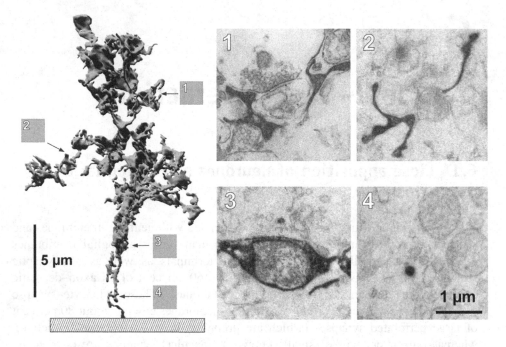

Figure 6.1 Close morphological contacts between Bergmann glial cells and Purkinje neurones in cerebellum. Left panel shows a three-dimensional reconstruction of an appendage extending from the process of the Bergmann glial cell. Electron micrographs of four sections contributing to the reconstruction (designated 1–4) are shown on the right; glial compartments appear black (from the injected dye). The location of these sections in the reconstruction is indicated by the labelled arrows. (1) Region directly contacting synapses. (2) Glial compartments without direct synaptic contacts. (3) Bulging glial structure containing a mitochondrion. (4) The stalk of the appendage. Note how completely the glial membranes enwrap the synaptic terminal in panel (1). (Modified from Grosche J, Matyash V, Moller T, Verkhratsky A, Reichenbach A, Kettenmann H (1999) Microdomains for neuron–glia interaction: parallel fiber signaling to Bergmann glial cells. *Nat Neurosci* **2**, 139–143)

cells express glutamate and purinoreceptors, whereas in the basal ganglia neurones and astrocytes are sensitive to dopamine. In the ability to sense neurotransmitter release, therefore, the astroglial cell closely resembles the postsynaptic neurone.

The close morphological relations between astrocytes and synapses as well as functional expression of relevant receptors in the astroglial cells prompted the appearance of a new concept of synaptic organization known as the 'tripartite synapse'. According to this concept, synapses are built from three equally important parts, the presynaptic terminal, the postsynaptic neuronal membrane and the surrounding astrocyte (Figure 6.2). Neurotransmitter released from the presynaptic terminal activates receptors in both the postsynaptic neuronal membrane and the perisynaptic astroglial membranes. This results in the generation of a postsynaptic potential in the neurone and a Ca^{2+} signal in the astrocyte. The latter may prop-

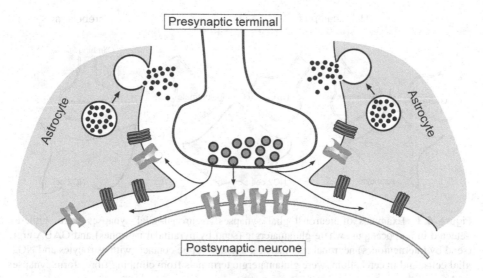

Figure 6.2 The tripartite synapse. The concept of the tripartite synapse assumes that it is constructed from a presynaptic terminal, the postsynaptic neuronal membrane, and surrounding astrocyte processes. The neurotransmitter released from the presynaptic terminal interacts with specific receptors located in both the postsynaptic neuronal membrane and in the astroglial membrane. Astrocytes may signal back to neurones by releasing 'gliotransmitters'

agate through the astroglial cell body or through astrocytic syncytium; this Ca^{2+} signal may also trigger release of 'glio' transmitters from astrocytes, which in turn will signal onto both pre- and postsynaptic neuronal membrane.

This concept of the tripartite synapse, which predicts bi-directional neuronal glial communication, has received strong experimental support, as both neurone-to-glia and glia-to-neurone signalling can be observed in the nervous system.

6.2   Neuronal–glial synapses

Direct synaptic contacts between neuronal terminals and both NG2-glia and astrocytes have been identified in hippocampus and cerebellum (Figure 6.3). Two types of neuronal–glial synapses, the excitatory glutamatergic synapses and the inhibitory GABAergic, formed by the terminals of pyramidal neurones and interneurones respectively, were recently detected in the hippocampus. These synapses have a typical morphology, revealed by electron microscopy; the latter shows axon terminals, filled with neurotransmitter-containing vesicles, which make synaptic junctions with the processes of glial cells. The neuronal–glial synapses are fully functional, as electric stimulation of nerve axons triggers neurotransmitter release and activation of the AMPA-type glutamate and $GABA_A$ receptors residing in the glial membrane. In the cerebellum, NG2-glia receive glutamatergic innervations

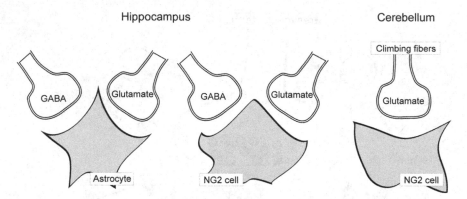

Figure 6.3 Examples of neuronal–glial synapses. Neuronal–glial synapses were, hitherto, detected in hippocampus, where glutamatergic (send by pyramidal neurones) and GABA-ergic (send by interneurones) neuronal terminals establish synaptic contacts with astrocytes and NG2-glial cells; and in cerebellum, were glutamatergic terminals from climbing fibres form synapses on NG2-glia

from climbing fibres; the terminals of the latter form numerous (up to 70) synaptic junctions on the processes of the glial cell.

6.3 Signalling from neurones to astrocytes

Stimulation of neurones or neuronal afferents triggers Ca^{2+} signalling in astrocytes both in cell cultures and *in situ* in brain slices. Moreover, astroglial cells are able to distinguish the intensity of neuronal activity. Astroglial Ca^{2+} oscillations induced by neuronal stimulation are clearly frequency encoded, the frequency increasing following an increase in synaptic activity. For example, it was found that astrocytes in hippocampus were able to follow the frequency of stimulation of neuronal afferents. The low frequency stimulation of neuronal fibres (the so-called Schaffer collaterals, through which neurones in the CA3 area are synaptically connected with neurones in the CA1 region) did not evoke any responses in astrocytes surrounding the synaptic terminals. High frequency stimulation, however, evoked repetitive Ca^{2+} signals in astrocytes, and the frequency of astroglial $[Ca^{2+}]_i$ elevations was directly dependent on the frequency or intensity of stimulation – increases in either led to a more frequent astrocytic response. Importantly, the Ca^{2+} responses in astrocytic processes were asynchronous, indicating the existence of relatively isolated compartments, able to follow activation of single synapses or small groups of synapses surrounded by a particular process. Similar to neurones, astrocytes also display cellular memory: periods of intense synaptic stimulation induce a long-lasting potentiation of the frequency of the subsequent responses (Figure 6.4). This phenomenon indeed resembles the long-term potentiation (LTP) of synaptic activity in neurones, in which intense synaptic stimulation

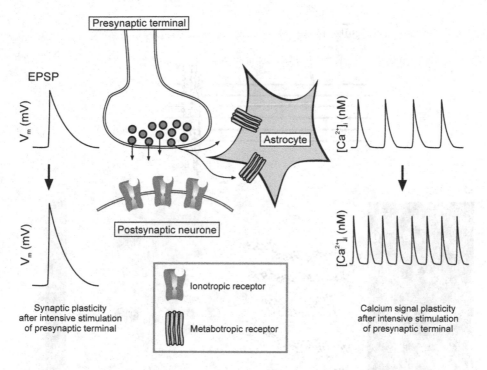

Figure 6.4 Long-term plasticity of astroglial Ca^{2+} signals. Astroglial Ca^{2+} signals undergo a long-term plasticity following periods of intense stimulation of presynaptic inputs, in a manner similar to neuronal postsynaptic electrical responses. The scheme shows a central glutamatergic synapse. Electrical stimulation of the terminal triggers excitatory postsynaptic potentials (EPSPs) in the neurone and Ca^{2+} signals in glial processes surrounding the synapse. Intense stimulation of synaptic inputs results in a long-term increase in the amplitude of the EPSP in the postsynaptic neurone (the phenomenon known as long-term potentiation, LTP), and in astrocytes results in a long-term increase in the frequency of glial Ca^{2+} responses. (Modified from Carmignoto G (2000) Reciprocal communication systems between astrocytes and neurones. *Prog Neurobiol* **62**, 561–581)

induces a long-lasting increase in the amplitude of post-synaptic potentials. The only difference between neurones and glia is in the parameter under regulation: in neurones this is the amplitude of the response, whereas in astrocytes it is the frequency.

A similar organization of glial responses to activation of neuronal afferents was also observed in Bergmann glial cells in the cerebellum. Fine processes of Bergmann glia enwrap synaptic terminals formed by parallel fibres on dendrites of Purkinje neurones. Stimulation of these parallel fibres resulted in highly localized Ca^{2+} signals in the processes of Bergmann glial cells (Figure 6.5), once more indicating the existence of relatively independent signalling microdomains, which can be individually activated by release of neurotransmitter from closely associated synaptic terminals.

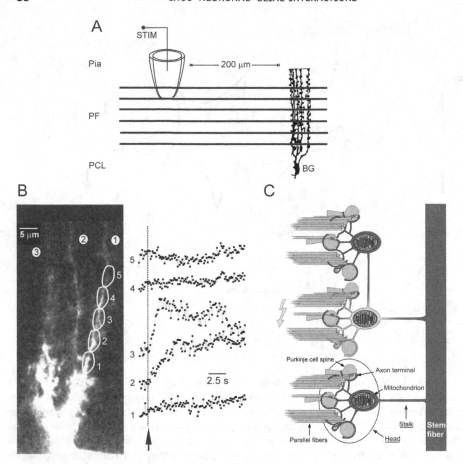

Figure 6.5 Localized intracellular Ca^{2+} signals in processes of Bergmann glial cells in response to synaptic activity:

A. Experimental protocol. Parallel fibres (PF) were stimulated via a pipette connected to a stimulator (STIM) while calcium-dependent fluorescence responses were recorded in a Bergmann glial cell (BG); PCL, Purkinje cell layer.

B. The left panel shows a confocal fluorescence intensity image of a patch-clamped Bergmann glial cell dialyzed with a calcium-sensitive dye (Oregon green 488 BAPTA-1). Three processes were distinguished (indicated as ①–③). Calcium signals in response to PF stimulation were measured independently in each process. The responding process (①) was subdivided into five regions of interest (marked 1–5), in which calcium signals were measured separately (middle panel; time of PF stimulation marked by an arrow and a dotted line).

C. Schematic representation of a Bergmann glial microdomain. The basic components of the microdomain, the stalk and the 'head', are shown together with their relationships to the neighbouring neuronal elements. Stimulation of several closely positioned parallel fibres may activate a single microdomain, inducing both membrane currents and local Ca^{2+} signals. (Modified from Grosche J, Matyash V, Moller T, Verkhratsky A, Reichenbach A, Kettenmann H (1999) Microdomains for neuron–glia interaction: parallel fiber signaling to Bergmann glial cells. *Nat Neurosci* **2,**139–143; and from Grosche J, Kettenmann H, Reichenbach A (2002) Bergmann glial cells form distinct morphological structures to interact with cerebellar neurons. *J Neurosci Res* **68,** 138–149)

6.4 Signalling from astrocytes to neurones

Calcium signals, which occur in astroglial cells either spontaneously or in response to activation of neighbouring neurones, are capable of triggering the release of neurotransmitters from the glial cells (see Chapter 5.6). It is now firmly established that these 'glio' transmitters can directly affect the neurones residing in the vicinity of the glial cells. This glial to neurone signalling is mediated by either ionotropic or metabotropic receptors present in the neuronal membrane. In particular, astroglial release of glutamate can directly depolarize (and hence excite) neurones through ionotropic glutamate receptors of AMPA and NMDA types. Glutamate can also activate metabotropic receptors residing in presynaptic terminals. Astrocytes can also modulate neuronal excitability through the release of ATP; the latter acting either directly, through stimulation of neuronal purinoreceptors, or indirectly, by degrading to adenosine and activating adenosine receptors.

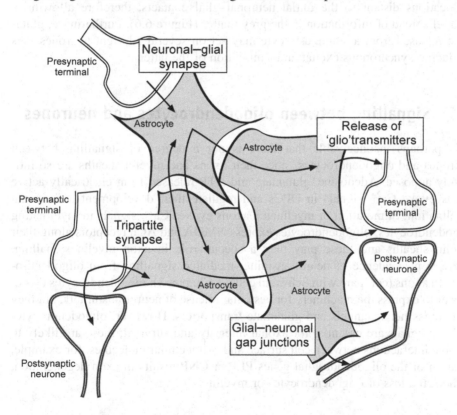

Figure 6.6 An overview of neuronal–glial interactions in the grey matter; scheme indicating the way in which reciprocal neuronal–glial communication may occur. Neurotransmitters released at 'neurone–glial' and 'tripartite' synapses act on astrocytes, to initiate Ca^{2+} signals that are propagated from astrocyte to astrocyte via gap junctions and the release of gliotransmitters, which in turn can act on distant synapses. In addition, signals may be communicated via glial–neuronal gap junctional contacts

Signalling from astrocytes to neurones has been demonstrated in a number of preparations, and it has been shown that neurotransmitters released from astrocytes can modulate neuronal activity. However, the significance of astrocyte–neuronal signalling in the integrative activity of the brain is at present speculative. Nonetheless, the machinery is present. It is clear that the release of glutamate from astrocytes is regulated by the frequency of Ca^{2+} oscillations – each single $[Ca^{2+}]_i$ peak triggers a pulsatile release of glutamate. Since the frequency of astroglial Ca^{2+} oscillations is governed by the intensity of synaptic activity, then an increase in the latter would substantially increase glutamate secretion from astrocytes, which would strengthen and amplify the original synaptic signal. Moreover, astrocytes release glutamate not only into the synaptic cleft, but elsewhere, which would induce activation of extrasynaptic receptors, which in turn could affect neuronal processing of incoming information. Finally, glial Ca^{2+} oscillations are conveyed through the astroglial network, which could induce the release of neurotransmitter in locations distant to the initial neuronal–glial contacts, therefore allowing a parallel spread of information in the grey matter (Figure 6.6). Furthermore, glutamate released from a single astrocyte may act on several adjacent neurones thus producing synchronous excitation or inhibition of the latter.

6.5 Signalling between oligodendrocytes and neurones

It is perhaps inconceivable that there is not a degree of signalling between neurones and oligodendrocytes, since their axons and myelin sheaths are so intimately apposed. Adenosine, glutamate and ATP released from electrically active axons evoke Ca^{2+} signals in OPCs and regulate their development and axonal myelination. Stimulation of myelinated axons evokes Ca^{2+} signals in myelinating oligodendrocytes; oligodendrocytes express NMDA and ACh receptors along their myelin sheaths and these may play a special role in axon–myelin signalling. There is no evidence of neurotransmitter-mediated signalling from oligodendrocytes to axons (compare with Schwann cells in Chapter 8): oligodendrocytes do not appear to express the machinery for vesicular release of neurotransmitters, but they do express hemichannels and glutamate transporters. However, oligodendrocyte-derived signals are essential for axonal integrity and survival; these are likely to involve interactions between cell surface and extracellular molecules; for example, ablation of the oligodendroglial genes PLP or CNP results in axon degeneration, without the loss of oligodendrocytes or myelin.

6.6 Signalling between Schwann cells and peripheral nerves and nerve endings

The perisynaptic Schwann cells are intimately integrated into the majority of vertebrate neuromuscular junctions. The processes of perisynaptic Schwann cells are closely associated with nerve terminals and send finger-like extensions directly into the synaptic cleft where they terminate very closely to the active zones. Similar to astrocytes, perisynaptic Schwann cells utilize intracellular Ca^{2+} as the substrate of their excitation. High-frequency stimulation of nerve terminals triggers $[Ca^{2+}]_i$ elevation in neighbouring Schwann cells. These $[Ca^{2+}]_i$ responses are mediated by neurotransmitters, as perisynaptic Schwann cells are endowed with metabotropic acetylcholine, ATP and substance P receptors, linked to Ca^{2+} release from the ER via the $InsP_3$ second messenger system. The Ca^{2+} signals generated in Schwann cells underlie the feedback to the neuronal terminal, as they can either potentiate or depress the release of neurotransmitters from the latter. The net effect (potentiation vs. depression) seems to be regulated by the frequency of synaptic activation.

PART II

Glial Cells and Nervous System Function

7
Astrocytes

Astroglial cells are truly multipotent and serve a surprizingly large and diverse variety of functions. These functions are absolutely vital for brain development, physiology and pathology.

Conceptually astroglial functions can be divided into several important groups:

Functions of astroglia

1. Developmental

   - Regulation of neuro and gliogenesis – astroglia are stem elements of the CNS.
   - Neuronal path finding.
   - Regulation of synaptogenesis.

2. Structural

   - Astroglia form the scaffold of the nervous system, thus defining the functional architecture of the brain and spinal cord.
   - Astrocytes form a continuous syncytium and integrate other neural cells into this syncytium.

3. Vascular – formation and regulation of the blood–brain barrier

   - Formation of the glial–vascular interface.
   - Regulation of cerebral microcirculation.

4. Metabolic

   - Providing energy substrates for neurones.
   - Collecting neuronal waste.

5. Control of the CNS microenvironment

   - Regulation of extracellular ion concentrations; in particular sequestration and redistribution of K^+ following fluctuations associated with neuronal activity.
   - Regulation of extracellular pH.

Glial Neurobiology: A Textbook Alexei Verkhratsky and Arthur Butt
© 2007 John Wiley & Sons, Ltd   ISBN 978-0-470-01564-3 (HB); 978-0-470-51740-6 (PB)

- Removal of neurotransmitters from the extracellular space.
- Brain water homeostasis.

6. Signalling

- Modulation of synaptic transmission.
- Release of neurotransmitters.
- Long-range signalling within the glial syncytium.
- Integration of neuronal–glial networks.

These functions are explained in more detail below.

7.1   Developmental function – producing new neural cells

7.1.1   Neurogenesis in the adult brain

In many vertebrates, neurogenesis persists throughout adulthood throughout the CNS. For example, new neurones are continuously born in all brain regions in birds, whilst lizards can very effectively regenerate the retina and spinal cord. In primates, including humans, neurogenesis in the adult is restricted to the hippocampus and subventricular zone. In both locations, the stem elements that produce neurones are astroglia. These 'stem' astrocytes have the morphology, physiology and biochemical/immunological markers characteristic for astrocytes: they express GFAP, form vascular endfeet, have negative resting membrane potentials, are nonexcitable, and predominantly express K^+ channels. 'Stem' astrocytes differ from 'classical' mature astrocytes by specific expression of the protein nestin (a marker for neural stem cells), and some of them form cilia. Neurones born in the subventricular zone migrate to the olfactory bulb, whereas those produced in the hippocampus remain there and integrate themselves into existing neuronal networks.

'Stem' astrocytes residing in the hippocampus and subventricular zone are multipotent, as they give birth to both neurones and glia; the production of glia or neurones is under control of numerous chemical factors (Figure 7.1).

7.1.2   Gliogenesis in adult brain

In the adult brain, in contrast to neurogenesis, gliogenesis occurs everywhere. New glial cells are born locally; and the locality also mainly determines the type of glial cell produced. In the subcortical white matter most of the newly produced glial cells are oligodendrocytes, whereas in the spinal cord astrocytes and oligodendrocytes are produced roughly in the same quantities.

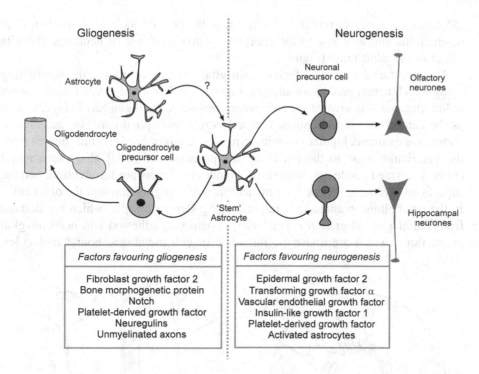

Gliogenesis | Neurogenesis

Astrocyte

Neuronal
precursor cell

Olfactory
neurones

Oligodendrocyte

Oligodendrocyte
precursor cell

'Stem'
Astrocyte

Hippocampal
neurones

Factors favouring gliogenesis	Factors favouring neurogenesis
Fibroblast growth factor 2 Bone morphogenetic protein Notch Platelet-derived growth factor Neuregulins Unmyelinated axons	Epidermal growth factor 2 Transforming growth factor α Vascular endothelial growth factor Insulin-like growth factor 1 Platelet-derived growth factor Activated astrocytes

Figure 7.1 Astrocytes as stem elements in the nervous system. In the adult CNS, 'stem' astrocytes can produce both neurones and glia. So far, it is almost impossible to distinguish between differentiated astrocytes and 'stem' astrocytes, and both retain mitotic potential. The precise pathways of transition of 'stem' astrocytes towards a glial or neuronal lineage are yet to be uncovered; however gliogenesis or neurogenesis can be promoted by various factors, some of which are listed

7.2   Developmental function – neuronal guidance

The vertebrate brain develops from the embryonic neuroectoderm that lies above the notochord and gives rise to the entire nervous system. The notochord induces neuroectodermal cells to generate neural stem cells and form the neural plate, which in turn forms the neural tube, from which the brain and spinal cord are derived. The neural precursor cells of the neural tube give rise to both neurones and glia in response to multiple inductive signals produced by the notochord, floor plate, roof plate, dorsal ectoderm and somites; for example, retinoic acid, fibroblast growth factor, bone morphogenetic proteins and sonic hedgehog. Inductive signals regulate transcription factors and gene expression, including the homeobox (Hox) genes, which influence the development of the neural tube into the major brain regions; forebrain (prosencephalon), midbrain (mesencephalon), and hindbrain (rhombencephalon). The first neural cells to develop are radial glia. After this, neural precursors in the ventricular zone (VZ) and subventricular zone

(SVZ) immediately surrounding the lumen of the neural tube migrate to their final destinations and give rise to the enormously diverse range of neurones and glia found in the adult brain (Figure 7.2).

An important function of foetal radial glial cells is to provide the scaffolding along which neural precursors migrate (Figure 7.2). Not all neurones migrate along radial glia, but it is always the case where neurones are organized in layers, such as the cerebellum, hippocampus, cerebral cortex and spinal cord. In the cerebral cortex, for example, bipolar postmitotic neurones migrate several millimetres from the ventricular zone to the pia along the processes of radial glia; the cerebral cortex is formed inside out, whereby the innermost layers are formed first, and the superficial layers are formed later by neurones that migrate through the older cells. In the cerebellum, granule cells migrate along Bergmann glia, which are derived from radial glia. Migration depends on recognition, adhesion and neurone–glial interactions, which are under the influence of cell membrane bound molecules,

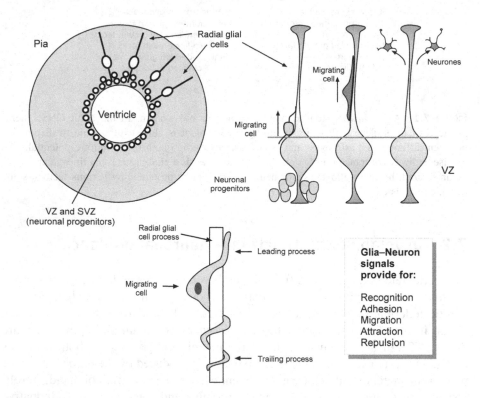

Figure 7.2 Radial glial cells form a scaffold that assists neuronal migration in the developing nervous system. Radial glial cells extend their processes from the ventricular zone (VZ) and subventricular zone (SVZ), where neural progenitors reside, towards the pia. Neuronal precursors attach to the radial glial cells and migrate along their processes towards their final destination. Numerous reciprocal factors released by both neurones and glia regulate the processes of mutual recognition, attraction, adhesion, migration and final repulsion

and diffusible and extracellular matrix molecules. Although the specific signals are not fully resolved, they include laminin–integrin interactions and neuregulin, which is expressed by migrating neurones and interacts with glial ErbB receptors. Subsequently, foetal radial glia disappear and transform into astrocytes; remnants of radial glia persist in the adult brain where they can generate olfactory and hippocampal neurones.

After neurones reach their final sites, they extend axons, which in some cases grow for considerable distances and have to cross the brain midline (decussate) to reach their synaptic targets. Channels formed by astrocytes provide a mechanical and guidance substrate for axon growth. In the corpus callosum, for example, astrocytes form a bridge (the glial sling) that connects left and right sides of the developing telencephalon. The ability of astrocytes to support axon growth decreases with age; embryonic astrocytes strongly support axon growth, whereas mature astrocytes inhibit axon growth – hence, the astroglial scar that forms following damage to the adult CNS is a major barrier to axon regeneration. Astrocytes produce a number of membrane bound and extracellular matrix molecules that serve as molecular cues for axon growth. These are generally considered to act by activating receptors on axonal growth cones to regulate process outgrowth; for example, N-cadherins and fibroblast growth factor receptors mediate neurite outgrowth by increased intracellular calcium in the growth cone. Astroglial laminin-1 is an excellent growth substrate for axons, and decussation of axons at the optic chiasm is dependent on laminin-1 and chondroitin sulphate proteoglycans produced at the glial boundary. Growth inhibitory molecules such as sempaphorins and ephrins also play important roles as guidance cues by regulating growth cone collapse.

7.3   Regulation of synaptogenesis and control of synaptic maintenance and elimination

The living brain constantly remodels and modifies its cellular networks. Throughout life, synapses continuously appear, strengthen, weaken or die. These processes underlie the adaptation of the brain to the constantly changing external environment and, in particular, represent what we know as learning and memory. For many years the process of synaptogenesis, maintenance and elimination of the synaptic contacts was considered to be solely neuronal responsibility; only very recently it has become apparent that glial cells (astrocytes in the CNS and Schwann cells in the PNS) control the birth, life and death of synapses formed in neuronal networks.

In general, the life cycle of the synapse proceeds through several stages: (1) formation of an initial contact between presynaptic terminal and postsynaptic neurone; (2) maturation of the synapse, when it acquires its specific properties, in particular the neurotransmitter modality; (3) stabilization and maintenance, which preserve the strong connections; and (4) elimination. In fact, the last stage may follow each of the preceding ones, and many synapses are eliminated before entering the stabilization phase.

The major wave of synaptogenesis in the mammalian brain starts shortly after birth, and lasts for several weeks in rodents and for a much longer period in humans. This wave of massive (as hundreds of billions of synapses have to occur within a relatively short time span) synaptogenesis precisely follows the massive generation of mature astrocytes, which happens during the perinatal period. This sequence of events is not coincidental as indeed astrocytes assist synapse appearance.

Synaptogenesis may occur in purified neuronal cultures, albeit at a relatively low rate; addition of astrocytes into this culture system dramatically (about seven times) increases the number of synapses formed. This increase in synaptic formation strictly depends on cholesterol, produced and secreted by astrocytes; cholesterol serves most likely as a building material for new membranes, which appear during synaptogenesis; in addition, cholesterol may be locally converted into steroid hormones, which in turn can act as synaptogenic signals. Glial cells also affect synaptogenesis through signals influencing the expression of a specific protein, agrin, essential for synapse formation.

After new synapses are formed, astrocytes control their maturation through several signalling systems affecting the postsynaptic density. In particular, intro-duction of astrocytes into neuronal cell cultures boosts the size of post-synaptic responses by increasing the number of post-synaptic receptors and facilitating their clustering. In contrast, removal of astroglial cells from neuronal cultures decreases the number of synapses. In part, these effects are mediated by several soluble factors released by astrocytes, although direct contact between glial and neuronal membranes also exerts a clear influence (of yet unidentified nature) on synapse maturation. Several distinct soluble factors have been identified that are released by glial cells and affect synapse maturation. One of them is tumour necrosis factor α (TNFα), which regulates the insertion of gluta-mate receptors into post-synaptic membranes; another one is activity-dependent neurotrophic factor (ADNF), which, after being secreted by astrocytes, increases the density of NMDA receptors in the membrane of neighbouring postsy-naptic neurones. In chick retina, Müller glial cells control the expression of M2 muscarinic ACh receptors in retinal neurones through a hitherto unidentified protein.

Astrocytes may also limit the number of synapses that appear on a given neurone, as astroglial membranes ensheathing the neurolemma prevent the forma-tion of new synaptic contacts. Astroglial cells can also be involved in the elimination of synapses in the CNS, the process which underlies the final tuning and plasticity of the neuronal inputs. This may be achieved by secretion of certain factors or proteolytic enzymes, which demolish the extracellular matrix and reduce the stability of the synaptic contact. Subsequently, astroglial processes may enter the synaptic cleft and literally close and substitute the synapse.

7.4 Structural function – creation of the functional microarchitecture of the brain

Protoplasmic astrocytes in the grey matter are organized in a very particular way, with each astrocyte controlling its own three-dimensional anatomical territory (Figure 7.3). The overlap between territories of neighbouring astroglial cells is minimal and it does not exceed five per cent, i.e. astrocytes contact each other only by the most distal processes. Individual astrocytes establish contacts with blood vessels, neurones and synapses residing within their anatomical domain. Astrocytic processes show a very high degree of morphological plasticity; many of these processes send very fine expansions, the lamellopodia and filopodia, which contact synaptic regions. These lamellopodia and filopodia are in fact motile, and may expand or shrink at a speed of several µm per minute. The lamellopodia show gliding movements along neuronal surfaces and filopodia are able to rapidly protrude towards or retract from the adjacent neuronal membranes or synaptic structures.

Using clearly delineated anatomical territories, astrocytes divide the whole of grey matter (both in the brain and in the spinal cord) into separate domains, the elements of which (neurones, synaptic terminals and blood vessels) are integrated via the processes of protoplasmic astrocytes; the membranes of a single astrocyte

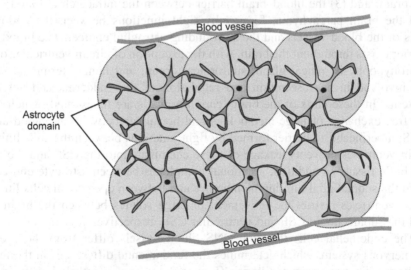

Figure 7.3 Astrocytic domains form the micro-architecture of grey matter. Each single astro-cyte occupies a well-defined territory; astroglial contacts occur only through distal processes and overall overlap between astrocyte territories does not exceed three to five per cent. The astrocytic domains are organized in rows along the vessels, which are typically positioned in the narrow interface between astrocytes as shown on the scheme. (Modified from Nedergaard M, Ransom B, Goldman SA (2003) New roles for astrocytes: redefining the functional architecture of the brain. *Trends Neurosci* **26,** 523–530)

may cover about 100 000 to 2 millions (in humans) synapses present in its domain. The astrocytic processes provide for local signalling within the domain, as their membranes that contact neurones, synapses and blood vessels are packed with receptors, which sense the ongoing activity. Signals activated by glial receptors may propagate through the astrocyte cytoplasm, thus integrating distant parts of the domain. Importantly, the processes of the same astrocyte are often directly coupled via gap junctions, which establish diffusion shortcuts, allowing the local metabolic signals to rapidly spread through these processes, bypassing the soma.

7.5 Vascular function – creation of glial–vascular interface (blood–brain barrier) and glia–neurone–vascular units

The brain tissue is separated from blood by three barrier systems: (1) the choroid plexus blood–CSF barrier in the ventricles of the brain, formed by tight junctions between the choroid plexus epithelial cells, which also produce the CSF; (2) the arachnoid blood–CSF barrier separating the subarachnoid CSF from the blood and formed by tight junctions between the cells of the arachnoid mater surrounding the brain; and (3) the blood–brain barrier between the intracerebral blood vessels and the brain parenchyma, formed by tight junctions between the endothelial cells of the blood vessels and the surrounding astroglial endfeet. The blood–brain barrier exists throughout the brain, with the exception of circumventricular organs, neurohypophysis, pineal gland, subfornical organ, and lamina terminalis, which are involved in neurosecretion and regulation of the endocrine and autonomic systems. In these parts of the brain, capillary walls are fenestrated, which allows the free exchange of large metabolites and hormones between the blood and the CNS; a permeability barrier formed by tight junctions between the cells lining the brain ventricles prevents leakage of these chemicals into the CSF and the rest of the brain tissue. In addition, junctional complexes between astrocyte endfeet that form the subpial glial limiting membranes and between ependymal cells lining the brain ventricles restrict the movement of large solutes between the brain tissue and the subarachnoid CSF and ventricular CSF, respectively.

The endothelial cells that line CNS blood vessels differ from those outside the nervous system, which determines the fundamental differences in the features of brain and non-brain capillaries (Figure 7.4). The endothelial cells in brain capillaries form numerous tight junctions, which effectively prevent paracellular transport of macromolecules or invasion of blood cells. In contrast, in nonneural capillaries the endothelial cells do not form continuous tight junctions; on the contrary the intercellular junctions are freely permeable to most solutes and in some cases capillaries have relatively large passages known as fenestrations, which allow paracellular diffusion of large molecular weight molecules and provide, when necessary, the pathway for infiltration of blood cells (i.e. macrophages) into the surrounding tissue.

From the brain side, the anatomical substrate of the blood–brain barrier is created by astroglial endfeet, which closely enwrap the capillary wall (Figure 7.4). The presence of an astroglial compartment around the blood vessels is of paramount importance for modifying the endothelial cells, as astrocytes release several regulatory factors (such as transforming growth factor α, TGFα, and glial-derived neurotrophic factor, GDNF), which induce the formation of tight junctions between endothelial cells and stimulate the polarization of their luminal and basal cell membranes (with respect to expression of various ion channels and proteins involved in transport across the blood–brain barrier). The endothelial cells, in turn also signal to astrocytes, in particular through leukaemia-inhibitory factor (LIF), which promotes astrocyte maturation. Contacts between astroglial endfeet and the endothelial cells also regulate expression of receptors and ion channels (especially aquaporins and K^+ channels) in the glial membrane.

The tight junctions between endothelial cells create the barrier between brain parenchyma and the circulation, essentially forming a sealed wall to the movement of even the smallest solutes (e.g. ions). The main function of this barrier is indeed

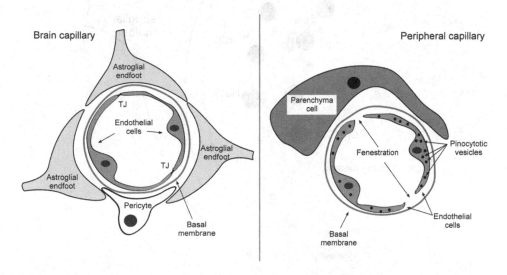

Figure 7.4 General structure of brain and peripheral capillaries. The scheme shows a cross-section of brain (CNS) and peripheral (systemic) capillaries. The endothelial cells of the brain capillary are sealed by tight junctions (TJ), which are the physical substrate of the blood–brain barrier and almost completely restrict diffusion of solutes between the blood and brain; hence, all solutes must pass through the endothelial cell (see Figure 7.5). Astroglial endfeet completely ensheath CNS capillaries and are important for induction and maintenance of blood–brain barrier properties and ion and water transport. In contrast, in peripheral blood vessels the intercellular junctions between endothelial cells are open and often fenestrated, and endothelial cells contain pinocytic vesicles, which are absent from most brain capillaries

to isolate the brain from the blood and provide a substrate for the brain's own homeostatic system. Everything that must cross the blood–brain barrier has to pass through the endothelial cells, which are selectively permeable to allow energy substrates and other essentials to enter, and metabolites to exit the brain tissue. The selective permeability is achieved by specific transporters residing in the endothelial cell membrane (Figure 7.5). These transporters are many and include (1) the energy-dependent adenine-nucleotide binding (ABC) cassette transporters, which excrete xenobiotics (this mainly determines the impermeability of the blood–brain barrier to many drugs, such as antibiotics, cytostatics, opioids etc.); (2) amino acid transporters; (3) glucose transporter of GLUT1 type; (4) ion exchangers etc.

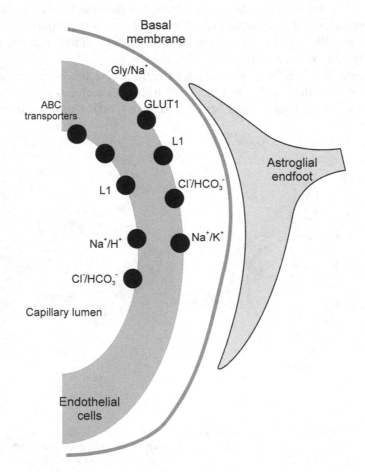

Figure 7.5 Transporter systems in the endothelial cell. The restricted permeability of the BBB means that essential solutes must be transported through the endothelial cells, which are endowed with numerous transport systems responsible for the exchange of essential solutes between blood and brain parenchyma, e.g. glucose and amino acids.

Abbreviations: ABC – adenine-nucleotide binding (ABC) cassette transporters; L1 –amino acid transporters; GLUT1 – glucose transporter; Na^+/H^+, Na^+/K^+, Cl^-/HCO_3^- – ion cotransporters

Many biologically active substances (e.g. catecholamines) cannot enter the brain precisely because the endothelial cells do not have the relevant transporters.

Astrocytes are not very much involved in blood–brain barrier function *per se* (which is determined largely by the endothelial cells), but astrocytes are important in the regulation of the blood–brain interface as a whole. Astrocyte endfeet membranes are enriched with numerous receptors, transporters and channels which mediate glial–endothelial communication and regulate exchange through the glial–vascular interface. In particular, endfeet are endowed with glucose transporters, which facilitate glucose uptake and its distribution to neurones (see below). The perivascular membranes of astrocyte end feet are also enriched in potassium channels (Kir4.1 subtype) and water channels (aquaporin-4 subtype), which are important for potassium and water transport at the blood–brain interface. It appears that all astrocytes participate in the glial–vascular interface (by at least one endfoot), through which the astrocyte maintains the exchange between blood and its own territory, thus establishing metabolically independent glia–neurone–vascular units (see Figure 7.3). Astrocytes also play a central role in regulation of the local vascular tone, hence linking the metabolic demands of grey matter with local blood supply.

7.6 Regulation of brain microcirculation

Increase in brain activity is tightly linked to the circulation, and local stimulation of neurones triggers a rapid increase in local blood flow. This phenomenon, known as *functional hyperaemia*, was discovered by Sherrington in 1890. Functional hyperaemia is a local phenomenon as vasodilatation occurs in small vessels within ~200–250 µm from the site of increased neuronal activity. Mechanisms of functional hyperaemia remained enigmatic for a long time; several hypotheses highlighted the role of local release of vasoactive factors, local innervation, or activation of nitric-oxide synthase and generation of NO. Recently, however, the crucial role of astroglia in control of microcirculation was identified.

The notion that astroglial cells provide a metabolic connection between neurones and blood vessels was initially made by Camillo Golgi in the 1870s. Recent advances in *in situ* cellular imaging have clearly demonstrated that astroglial Ca^{2+} signals triggered by neuronal activity enter endfeet and initiate the release of vasoactive substances, which in turn affect the tone of small arterioles enwrapped by these endfeet. Inhibition of astroglial Ca^{2+} signalling inhibits the functional link between neuronal activation and changes in vascular tone. In fact, astrocytes are able to provide dual control over the neighbouring blood vessels: they may either induce vasodilatation or vasoconstriction. Interestingly both effects begin with Ca^{2+} elevation in the endfeet and the release of arachidonic acid (AA). The latter can be transformed into prostaglandin derivatives by cyclo-oxygenase (COX), which can be blocked by aspirin; these derivatives of AA effectively relax the vascular muscle cells and cause vasodilatation and increased blood flow.

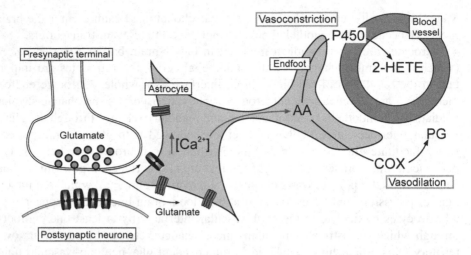

Figure 7.6 Model for astroglial-dependent regulation of local blood flow – astroglial cells couple neuronal activity with local circulation by releasing vasoconstrictors and vasodilators: Glutamate released at synapses during increased neuronal activity activates calcium signals in astrocytic processes enwrapping synaptic contacts. Calcium signals propagate through the astroglial cell (and astroglial syncytium) to reach the perivascular endfoot, where Ca^{2+} triggers the release of arachidonic acid (AA). Depending on the brain region and local enzymatic systems, AA can be converted to vasodilatatory prostaglandins (PG) by cyclo-oxygenase (COX), or to a vasoconstrictive agent 20 hydroxyeicosatetraenois acid (2-HETE), by a cytochrome P450 epoxygenase of the arteriole smooth muscle

Alternatively, AA can be converted into the vasoconstrictive agent 20 hydroxyeicosatetraenois acid (2-HETE) by a cytochrome 450 enzyme residing in the arteriole smooth muscle (Figure 7.6).

7.7 Ion homeostasis in the extracellular space

Maintenance of the extracellular ion composition is of paramount importance for brain function, because every shift in ion concentrations profoundly affects the membrane properties of nerve cells and hence their excitability. Brain extracellular space contains high amounts of Na^+ ($[Na^+]_o \sim 130$ mM) and Cl^- ($[Cl^-]_o \sim 100$ mM), whereas it is rather low in K^+ ($[K^+]_o \sim 2$–2.5 mM). This is reversed inside the brain cells, as the cytosol of most of neurones and glia is rich in K^+ ($[K^+]_i \sim 100$–140 mM) and poor in Na^+ ($[Na^+]_i \sim <10$ mM). The intracellular chloride concentration is, as a rule, low in neurones ($[Cl^-]_i \sim 2$–10 mM) and is relatively high in glial cells ($[Cl^-]_i \sim 30$–35 mM), due to Cl^- influx in exchange for Na^+ and K^+ by the $Na^+/K^+/Cl^-$ transporters. The extracellular concentration of another important cation, Ca^{2+}, is relatively low in the extracellular space ($[Ca^{2+}]_o \sim 1.5$–2 mM), nevertheless it is still about 20 000 times lower in the cytosol ($[Ca^{2+}]_i \sim 0.0001$ mM). These transmembrane ion gradients together with selective plasmalemmal ion channels form the basis for generation and maintenance of the resting membrane potential and underlie neuronal excitability. The safeguarding of transmembrane ion gradients is the task for numerous ion-transporting systems, which allow ion movements either by diffusion (ion channels) or at the expense of energy (ion pumps and exchangers). The main ion transporters operative in astrocytes are summarized in Figure 7.7.

Apart from preserving their own transmembrane ion homeostasis, astroglial cells are heavily involved in maintenance of extracellular ion concentrations. As neuronal activity is inevitably associated with influx of Na^+ and Ca^{2+} (depolarization) and efflux of K^+ (repolarization), the extracellular concentrations of these ions vary; the relative variations are especially high for K^+ ions (due to a low $[K^+]_o$ and a very limited volume of the CNS extracellular space; i.e. even relatively modest numbers of K^+ ions released by neurones may very substantially affect the extracellular K^+ concentration). If the K^+ released during action potential propagation was allowed to accumulate in the extracellular space, this would cause neuronal depolarization. Small increases in $[K^+]_o$ would increase neuronal excitability by bringing their membrane potential closer to the action potential threshold. If K^+ rises sufficiently to depolarize the neurones past the threshold

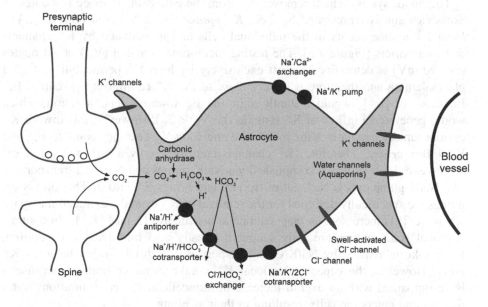

Figure 7.7 Ion transporting systems in the astroglial cell. The main astroglial ion transporters are: Na^+/H^+ antiporter; $Na^+/H^+/HCO_3^-$ and $Na^+/K^+/2Cl^-$ cotransporters; Cl^-/HCO_3^- and Na^+/Ca^{2+} exchangers; Na^+/K^+ pumps; water channels (aquaporins); K^+ and Cl^- channels and swell-activated Cl^- channels. Glia also contain carbonic anhydrase, which catalyzes the conversion of $H_2O + CO_2$ to carbonic acid (H_2CO_3), which readily dissociates to H^+ and HCO_3^-, hence facilitating CO_2 uptake and extracellular pH regulation during neuronal activity

for Na^+ channel activation, neurones become inexcitable because Na^+ channels become inactivated and there is a conduction block. Astrocytes help prevent the accumulation of extracellular K^+, thereby stabilizing neuronal activity.

7.7.1 Astrocytes and extracellular potassium homeostasis

During intense (but still physiological) neuronal activity the extracellular potassium concentration may rise almost twice, from 2–2.5 mM to 4–4.2 mM; such an increase can be observed, for example, in the cat spinal cord during rhythmic and repetitive flexion/extension of the knee joint. As a rule, however, during regular physiological activity in the CNS the $[K^+]_o$ rarely increases by more than 0.2 to 0.4 mM. Nonetheless, locally, in tiny microdomains such as for instance occurring in narrow clefts between neuronal and astroglial membranes in perisynaptic areas, $[K^+]_o$ may transiently attain much higher levels. The relatively small rises in $[K^+]_o$ accompanying physiological neuronal activity indicate that powerful mechanisms controlling extracellular potassium are in operation. Disruption of these mechanisms, which do occur in pathology, results in a profound $[K^+]_o$ dyshomeostasis; upon epileptic seizures, for example, $[K^+]_o$ may reach 10–12 mM, while during brain ischaemia and spreading depression $[K^+]_o$ can transiently peak at 50–60 mM.

The major system which removes K^+ from the extracellular space is located in astrocytes and is represented by *local K^+ uptake* and *K^+ spatial buffering*. The *local K^+ uptake* occurs in the individual cells and is mediated by K^+ channels and transporters (Figure 7.8). The resting membrane potential (V_m) of astrocytes ($\sim$ –90 mV) is determined almost exclusively by high K^+ permeability of glial plasmalemma and therefore it is very close to the K^+ equilibrium potential, E_K. Increases in $[K^+]_o$ would instantly shift the E_K towards depolarization, which would generate an inflow of K^+ ions (as the $V_m < E_K$). However, this inward K^+ current rapidly depolarizes the membrane and soon V_m becomes equal to E_K, and K^+ influx ceases. Therefore, K^+ channels contribute only a little towards local K^+ uptake. Most of it is accomplished via Na/K pumps and Na/K/Cl transporters. The Na/K pump expels Na^+ out of the cell and brings K^+ into it. The glial Na/K pumps are specifically designed for the removal of K^+ from the extracellular space when $[K^+]_o$ is increased, as they saturate at around 10–15 mM $[K^+]_o$; in contrast neuronal Na/K pumps are fully saturated already at 3 mM $[K^+]_o$. In addition, K^+ uptake is assisted by Na/K/Cl cotransport, in which Cl^- influx balances K^+ entry. However, the capacity for local K^+ uptake is rather limited, because it is accompanied with an overall increase in intracellular K^+ concentration; water follows and enters the cells, resulting in their swelling.

A much more powerful and widespread mechanism for the removal of excess extracellular K^+ is *spatial buffering*, a model proposed in the 1960s by Wolfgang Walz and Richard Orkand. In this case, K^+ ions entering a single cell are redistributed throughout the glial syncytium by intercellular K^+ currents through gap junctions. After this spatial redistribution, K^+ ions are expelled into either the

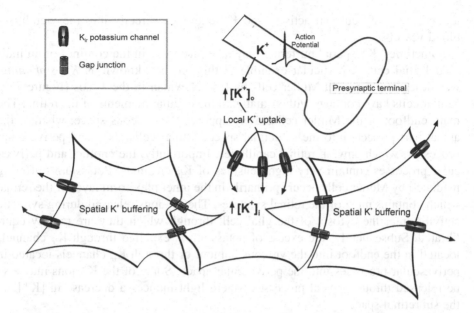

Figure 7.8 Astrocytes provide for local and spatial potassium buffering: Buffering of extracellular potassium occurs through astroglial inward rectifier potassium channels K_{ir} (local potassium buffering). Potassium is released into the extracellular space during neuronal activity (K^+ efflux underlies the recovery phase – repolarization – of the action potential). Astrocytes take up excess K^+ through K_{ir}, redistribute the K^+ through the astroglial syncytium via gap junctions (spatial potassium buffering), and release K^+ through K_{ir}. See the text for further details

interstitium or perivascular space, where they are removed into the blood. In spatial, K^+ buffering, the K^+ ions are transported across the membranes through K^+ channels. Local K^+ entry depolarizes the cell, which creates an electrical and chemical gradient between this cell and neighbouring astrocytes connected via gap junctions. This provides the force for K^+ ions to diffuse into the syncytium, preventing local membrane depolarization (thus maintaining K^+ influx) and dispersing K^+ ions through many cells, so that the actual elevation in cytoplasmic K^+ concentration is minimal (Figure 7.8). The principal K^+ channels responsible for spatial buffering are inwardly rectifying channels of $K_{ir}4.1$ type. These channels are only mildly rectifying; i.e. they allow both inward and outward K^+ movements at the resting membrane potential levels. This is important, as K^+ is finally expelled from the glial syncytium also through the K_{ir} channels. Another important feature of K_{ir} channels is that their conductance is directly regulated by the $[K^+]_o$ levels; the conductance increases as a square root of increase in $[K^+]_o$. In other words, local increases in $[K^+]_o$ augments the rate of K^+ accumulation of glial cells. The K_{ir} channels are clustered in perisynaptic processes of astroglial cells and in their endfeet (where the density of K_{ir} channels can be up to 10 times larger that in the rest of the cell membrane). This peculiar distribution facilitates K^+ uptake around areas of neuronal activity and K^+ extrusion directly into the vicinity of blood vessels.

Sometimes, K^+ spatial buffering may take place within the confines of an individual glial cell. A particular example of this process, known as *K^+ siphoning*, was described in retinal Müller cells by Eric Newman in the 1980s (Figure 7.9). Müller cells have contacts with virtually all the cellular elements of the retina. The main endfoot of the Müller cell closely apposes the vitreous space, whereas the apical part projects into the subretinal space; Müller cells also send perivascular processes, which enwrap retinal capillaries. Importantly, the endfoot and perivascular processes contain very high densities of K_{ir} channels. Potassium buffering mediated by Müller cells occurs primarily in the inner plexiform layer of the retina, which contains most of the retinal synapses. The K^+ ions released during synaptic activity enter the cytosol of the glial cell, through which they are rapidly equilibrated. Subsequently, the excess of potassium is expelled through K_{ir} channels located in the endfoot into the vitreous humour or through K_{ir} channels located in perivascular processes into the perivascular space. Some of the K^+ ions may also be released through apical processes, where light induces a decrease in $[K^+]_o$ in the subretinal space.

7.7.2 Astrocytes and chloride homeostasis

Astrocytes contribute to overall chloride homeostasis by activation of anion channels. As the cytosolic concentration of Cl^- in astroglial cells is high, opening of anion channels will cause Cl^- efflux. This efflux is activated during hypo-osmotic stress. Alternatively astrocytes can accumulate chloride by $Na^+/K^+/2Cl^-$ cotransporter.

7.7.3 Astrocytes and extracellular Ca^{2+}

Calcium concentration in small extracellular compartments and particularly in perisynaptic compartments may fluctuate rather substantially, as Ca^{2+} is accumulated by neurones when the invading action potential activates Ca^{2+} channels. The actual $[Ca^{2+}]_o$ can decrease below 1 mM, which may affect generation of Ca^{2+} signals in the terminal, and hence neurotransmission. The lowering of extracellular Ca^{2+} concentration to ~0.5 mM triggers Ca^{2+} signalling in astrocytes, which originates from $InsP_3$-driven intracellular Ca^{2+} release from the ER stores. This may, in principle, help restore $[Ca^{2+}]_o$, as Ca^{2+} can leave the astrocyte through either plasmalemmal Ca^{2+} pump or sodium–calcium exchanger. Extracellular Ca^{2+} concentration may plunge much deeper (to 0.01–0.1 mM) under ischaemic conditions, which in turn can initiate seizures (see Chapter 10).

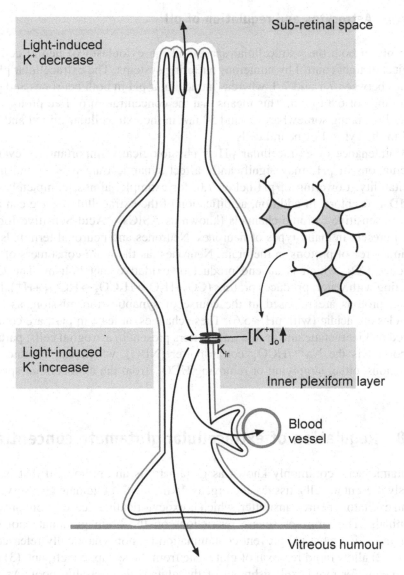

Figure 7.9 'Potassium siphoning' in retinal Müller glial cell. Potassium buffering in the retina is provided by Müller glial cells: K^+ ions enter the cytosol of the Müller cell in the inner plexiform layer; K^+ then equilibrates within the glial cytosol and excess K^+ is expelled through K_{ir} channels located in the endfoot into the vitreous humour or through K_{ir} channels located in perivascular processes into the perivascular space. Some of the K^+ ions may be also released through apical processes, where light induces a decrease in $[K^+]_o$ in the subretinal space. The same process of K^+ siphoning can occur in astrocytes, taking up K^+ via their perisynaptic or perinodal processes and releasing K^+ via their perivascular endfeet, where it could help regulate blood flow

7.7.4 Astrocytes and regulation of pH

The pH in both the extracellular space and the cytoplasm of neural cells is the subject of tight control by numerous buffering systems. The extracellular pH (pH_o) varies between 7.1 and 7.3, whereas intracellular pH in both neurones and glia lies in a range of 6.8 to 7.5. This means that the concentration of free protons, H^+, is quite low, being somewhere around 50 nM in the extracellular milieu and 30–160 nM in the cytosol of neural cells.

Maintenance of extracellular pH is physiologically important, as even small fluctuations of pH_o may significantly affect synaptic transmission and neuronal excitability. Lowering of pH below 7.0, for example, almost completely inhibits NMDA receptors; in addition, acidification of the extracellular space can activate proton-sensitive cationic channels (known as ASICs – Acid-Sensitive Ion Channels) present in many types of neurones. Neurones and neuronal terminals are the main source of protons in the brain. Neurones, as the main consumers of energy, produce CO_2, which is an end product of oxidative metabolism. The CO_2, by reacting with water, produces protons ($CO_2 + H_2O \leftrightarrow H_2CO_3 \leftrightarrow HCO_3^- + H^+$). Furthermore, protons are released in the course of synaptic transmission, as synaptic vesicles are acidic (with pH ~5.6). These changes, at least in part, are counterbalanced by bicarbonate and proton transporters present in astroglial cells; particularly important is the Na^+/HCO_3^- cotransporter (NBC), which can operate in both directions, either supplying or removing HCO_3^- from the extracellular space.

7.8 Regulation of extracellular glutamate concentration

Glutamic acid, commonly known as glutamate, is an amino acid that is ubiquitously present in cells, tissues and organs. In the CNS, glutamate also serves as the main excitatory neurotransmitter, which is exocytotically released from presynaptic terminals. This imposes severe restrictions on the brain glutamate homeostatic system, which must (1) prevent contamination by nonsynaptically released glutamate, (2) allow rapid removal of glutamate from the synaptic cleft, and (3) provide the means for rapid replenishment of the glutamate-releasable pool. As if these are not enough, background extracellular glutamate concentration should always be kept very low, as glutamate in excess is highly neurotoxic. Precise regulation of extracellular concentration of glutamate is, therefore, of paramount importance for brain function.

The first cornerstone of this regulation is laid by blood–brain barrier, which does not allow glutamate from the circulation to enter the CNS; as a consequence, all glutamate in the brain must be synthesized within the brain. A second important part of the glutamate homeostatic system is created by the specific morphological organization of glutamatergic synapses, which are often completely enclosed by the membrane of astrocytic perisynaptic processes; such an organization prevents glutamate from spilling over from the synaptic cleft and contaminating nearby synapses. Third, the glutamate in the synaptic cleft is very rapidly removed by glutamate transporters (see also Chapter 5.7), which are located either in astroglial membranes or in the postsynaptic neuronal membrane. The presynaptic terminal is devoid of glutamate transporters.

Astroglial cells represent the main sink of glutamate in the brain (Figure 7.10); from the bulk of glutamate released during synaptic transmission, about 20 per cent is accumulated into postsynaptic neurones and the remaining 80 per cent is taken up by perisynaptic astrocytes. Thus, synaptic transmission is associated with a continuous one-directional flow of glutamate into astroglial cells. Quite obviously, such a process would rapidly deplete the pool of releasable neurotransmitter. Astrocytes therefore have a special system for recovering glutamate to the presynaptic terminal. After being accumulated by astrocyte, glutamate is converted into glutamine, and it is this glutamine that is released by the astrocyte into the extracellular space for subsequent uptake into presynaptic neurones – the so-called *glutamate–glutamine shuttle* (Figure 7.10); as glutamine is physiologically inactive, its appearance in the extracellular milieu is harmless. Conversion of glutamate to glutamine is catalyzed by glutamine synthetase (highly expressed by astrocytes, and used as a specific marker) and requires energy (one ATP molecule

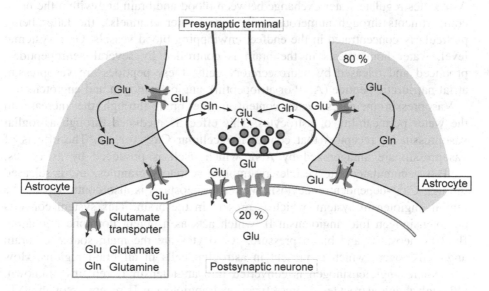

Figure 7.10 Glutamate uptake by glial and neuronal cells – the glutamate–glutamine shuttle. Glutamate released during synaptic activity is removed from the cleft by glutamate transporters; about 80 per cent of glutamate is accumulated by astrocytes and ~20 per cent by postsynaptic neurones; presynaptic terminals do not accumulate glutamate. After entering the astrocyte, glutamate is converted into glutamine, which is then transported back to the presynaptic terminal, where it is converted into glutamate and accumulated into synaptic vesicles. This recycling of glutamate by astrocytes is known as the glutamate–glutamine shuttle

per conversion); importantly glutamate uptake into astrocytes triggers glucose hydrolysis, which provides ATP, and links neuronal activity with the supply of energy substrates (see Chapter 7.10 for details). When glutamine enters the presynaptic neurone it is hydrolysed to glutamate; this process, which is assisted by phosphate-activated glutaminase, does not require energy. The newly synthesized glutamate is concentrated in synaptic vesicles, endowed with specific vesicular glutamate transporters. This is the endpoint for the glutamate–glutamine shuttle, which allows for sustained glutamatergic synaptic transmission.

Similarly important is the involvement of astroglial glutamate uptake in preventing excitotoxic accumulation of high glutamate levels in the extracellular space, and removal of astrocytes from neuronal glial co-cultures, for example, greatly increases neuronal vulnerability and amplifies neuronal death.

7.9 Water homeostasis and regulation of the extracellular space volume

7.9.1 Regulation of water homeostasis

Astrocytes regulate water exchange between blood and brain and within the brain compartments through numerous aquaporins (water channels), the latter being particularly concentrated in the endfeet enwrapping blood vessels. On a systemic level, water homeostasis in the brain is controlled by several neuropeptides, produced and released by neurosecretory cells; these peptides are vasopressin, atrial natriuretic peptide (ANP or atriopeptin), angiotensinogen and angiotensin.

Vasopressin increases water content in the brain through the increase in the water permeability of astrocytes. This effect is mediated through astroglial vasopressin V_1 receptors that control intracellular Ca^{2+} release. The effects of vasopressin are antagonized by ANP which itself is produced by astrocytes. ANP is accumulated into vesicles resembling secretory granules, and is released through Ca^{2+}-dependent exocytosis. Water homeostasis is also controlled by the rennin–angiotensin system, which is present in the brain. This system converts angiotensinogen into angiotensin II, which acts as a potent hormone regulating fluid homeostasis and blood pressure. Astrocytes are the main source of brain angiotensinogen, which is present in astroglial cells in all brain regions. How and where angiotensinogen is converted into angiotensin II remains unknown; although many astrocytes express functional angiotensin II receptors of the AT_1 type. Activation of these receptors causes intracellular Ca^{2+} release and secretion of prostacyclin from a subpopulation of astrocytes in the cerebellum and medulla.

Astrocytes are also able to sense changes in extracellular osmolarity. When the osmolarity of the extracellular milieu is decreased (hypo-osmotic stress), astrocytes rapidly swell; this swelling is followed by a so-called regulatory volume decrease (RVD), which corrects the initial increase in cell volume. RVD is a complex process, which involves extrusion of intracellular osmotically active substances, including K^+ and Cl^-, as well as some organic molecules, such as organic amines. Hypo-osmotic shock also triggers efflux of neurotransmitters glutamate, glycine, taurine and GABA. The precise mechanisms of RVD are not yet fully understood; a particular role may be played by volume(swell)-activated K^+ and Cl^- channels; the latter may also be permeable to glutamate and taurine. Release of taurine is especially important in the osmosensitive regions of the brain. In conditions of hypo-osmotic stress astrocytes in the supra-optic nucleus and in circumventricular organs release taurine, which activates glycine receptors of osmosensitive neurones.

7.9.2 Redistribution of water following neuronal activity and regulation of the extracellular space

High synaptic activity is associated with a transient decrease in the extracellular space surrounding the active synapses. This is physiologically important, as local restriction of the extracellular space modulates the efficacy of synaptic transmission by (1) increasing the local concentration of neurotransmitter, and (2) limiting the spillover of the transmitter from the synaptic cleft. This local shrinkage of the extracellular space following neuronal activity is regulated by water transport across astroglial membranes and water redistribution through the glial syncytium. Water accumulated at the site of high neuronal activity is released distantly, which causes an increase in extracellular volume. Such coordinated changes in extracellular volume have been directly observed, for example, in the cortex, where stimulation of neuronal afferents caused a local decrease in extracellular volume in layer IV and a simultaneous increase in the extracellular space in layer I. These changes in extracellular volume are directly coupled to the astroglial syncytium, as they can be eliminated following uncoupling of the glial cells by pharmacological inhibition of gap junctions.

This redistribution of water during neuronal activity is mediated through the aquaporins, which show a very special distribution across the astrocyte plasmalemma. Aquaporin channels (especially AQP4) are clustered in the perivascular and subpial endfeet and in perisynaptic processes and are colocalized with the $K_{ir}4.1$ channel subtype (Figure 7.11). Synaptic activity causes local elevations of extracellular concentrations of glutamate, K^+ and CO_2; glutamate and K^+ are accumulated by astrocytes through glutamate transporter and K_{ir} channels, respectively, whereas CO_2 is transported into the astrocyte via Na^+/HCO_3^- cotransporter. These events increase local osmotic pressure at the astrocyte membrane, which favours water intake through the aquaporins; removal of extracellular water leads to shrinkage of the extracellular space. Locally accumulated water is redistributed through the astroglial network and is extruded distantly (also through aquaporins) therefore increasing the extracellular volume near the place of efflux.

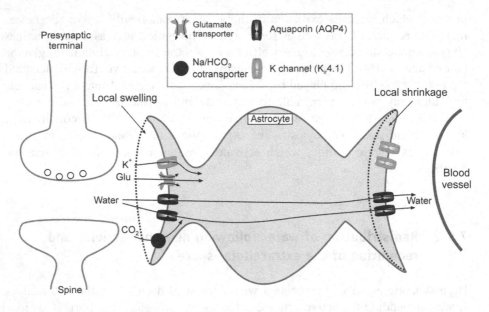

Figure 7.11 Water transport and neuronal-activity-dependent regulation of extracellular volume by astrocytes

This scheme of water redistribution following neuronal activity is equivalent to that of spatial K^+ buffering (Chapter 7.7.1), which suggested possible coordination between water and K^+ transport across astroglial membranes. This idea gained credibility recently, after direct coupling between aquaporins and K_{ir} channels ($K_{ir}4.1$) was discovered on a molecular level. Furthermore it appears that transgenic mice lacking aquaporins in the perivascular astrocytic processes also have an impaired spatial K^+ buffering.

7.10 Neuronal metabolic support

The brain produces energy by oxidizing glucose; the brain receives glucose and O_2 from the blood supply. Glucose is transported across the blood–brain barrier via glucose transporter type 1 (GLUT1), which is specifically expressed in endothelial cells forming the capillary walls. Following transport across the blood–brain barrier, glucose is released into the extracellular space and is accumulated by neural cells via more plasmalemmal glucose transporters (Figure 7.12); neurones predominantly express GLUT3, whereas astrocytes possess GLUT1. Upon entering the cells, glucose is oxidized through glycolysis and the tricarboxylic acid cycle (TCA or Krebs cycle), which are central steps in energy production. Neurones account for about 90 per cent of brain energy consumption, and glial cells are

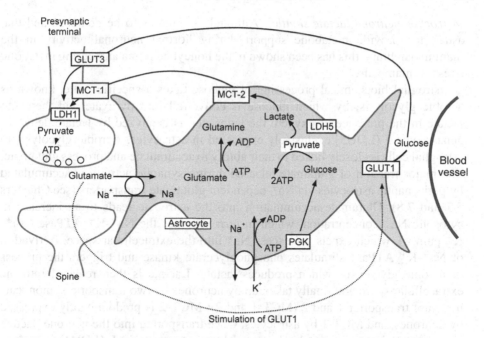

Figure 7.12 The 'astrocyte–neuronal lactate shuttle': a mechanism by which astrocytes can provide an energy substrate to active neurones. The scheme shows biochemical and physiological pathways that have been demonstrated in astrocytes and neurones. These provide the substrate of the astroglial–neuronal lactate shuttle, detailed explanations of which are given in the text. Astrocytes take up glucose (via GLUT1) and convert it pyruvate and then lactate (via LDH5). Glutamate released during neuronal activity is taken up by astrocytes and triggers them to release lactate (via MCT-2), which is subsequently taken up by the neurone (via MCT-1), which utilizes it as a metabolic substrate (via LDH1). This provides a mechanism for coupling neuronal activity and astrocyte metabolism.

Abbreviations: GLUT1 – astroglial glucose transporter type 1; GLUT3 – neuronal glucose transporter type 3; LDH1 and LDH5 – lactate dehydrogenase type 1 and 5; MCT-1 and MCT-2 monocarboxylase transporters 1 and 2

responsible for the remaining 10 per cent; neurones require a continuous supply of energy to fuel their Na^+-K^+ ATPases (Na^+-K^+ pumps), which are constantly active to maintain ion gradients across neuronal cell membranes in the face of the continuous ionic fluxes during synaptic activity and action potential propagation. However, monitoring the distribution of glucose in the brain tissue has demonstrated that it is accumulated equally by neurones and astroglial cells. This implies the involvement of an intermediate product of glucose utilization, which is produced by astrocytes and subsequently transported to neurones. Furthermore, the utilization of glucose by the brain strongly depends on neural activity, a process that can be readily demonstrated by functional brain imaging, for example, positron emission tomography.

It turns out that astrocytes are ideally situated and have the biochemical machinery to provide metabolic support for neurones via the so-called '*astrocyte–neurone lactate shuttle*'. Although it remains to be demonstrated that astrocytes provide metabolic support during normal neuronal activity in the mammalian brain, this has been shown in the honeybee retina and during metabolic stress in mammals.

Astroglial biochemical processing of glucose takes a specific route, known as aerobic glycolysis, by which glucose is converted into pyruvate and then into lactate in the presence of oxygen; the latter step is catalyzed by lactate dehydrogenase type 5 (LDH5) exclusively expressed in astrocytes. Aerobic glycolysis in astroglial cells is closely linked to their ability to accumulate and process glutamate. The major fraction of glutamate released during synaptic activity is accumulated by perisynaptic astrocytes via Na^+-dependent glutamate transporters (see Chapters 5.7 and 7.8). Glutamate accumulation into the astrocyte leads to an increase in cytosolic Na^+ concentration, which in turn activates the Na^+-K^+ ATPase (Na^+-K^+ pumps), which expels the excess Na^+ into the extracellular space. Activation of Na^+-K^+ ATPase stimulates phosphoglycerate kinase and triggers the process of aerobic glycolysis, which produces lactate. Lactate is then released into the extracellular space and finally taken up by neurones by two transporters, monocarboxylase transporter 1 and 2 (MCT-1 and 2); MCT-2 is predominantly expressed by neurones, and MCT-1 by astrocytes. Once transported into the neurone, lactate is converted into pyruvate by lactate dehydrogenase type 1 (LDH1), which is expressed in neurones (as well as other lactate-consuming tissues). Pyruvate enters the TCA cycle and is utilized to produce energy.

Thus, glutamate released in the course of synaptic transmission acts as a specific signal on astrocytes to increase their delivery of an energy supply to active nerve cells. Every molecule of glutamate taken up by the astrocyte brings with it three Na^+ ions. This activates Na^+/K^+ ATPase and aerobic glycolysis, which produces two molecules of ATP and two molecules of lactate from one molecule of glucose. The ATP so produced is consumed by Na^+/K^+ ATPase (one ATP molecule for expelling the three Na^+ ions accumulated from glutamate transport), and by glutamine synthetase (one ATP molecule is needed for conversion of one molecule of the accumulated glutamate into one molecule of glutamine). The resulting two molecules of lactate are transported to the neurone, where each lactate molecule, being processed through the TCA cycle, delivers 17 molecules of ATP. This process of activity-induced 'astrocyte–neurone lactate shuttle' is further assisted by specific stimulation of astroglial glucose transporters by glutamate, which rapidly (in $\sim$10 seconds) induces a two to three fold increase in astrocyte GLUT1-mediated glucose uptake.

Besides regulating the activity-dependent nourishment of neurones through the glucose–lactate shuttle, astrocytes also contain the brain reserve energy system. This system relies upon glycogen, which in the brain is present almost exclusively in astroglial cells. Glycogen is mobilized and turned into glucose upon intensive stimulation of the CNS. Subsequently, the glucose so-produced can be used by neurones (through the lactate shuttle), or by astrocytes themselves to meet high energy demands in response to intensive synaptic activity.

7.11   Astroglia regulate synaptic transmission

Astroglia affect neuronal synaptic transmission in several ways. First, astrocytes modulate synaptic strength by controlling the concentration of neurotransmitter in the cleft via glial transporters. This is the case for most synapses that use amino acid neurotransmitters, such as glutamate, GABA, and monoamines, where astrocytes express specific transporters, depending on the synapse (see Chapter 5.7). Alternative mechanisms of affecting neurotransmitter concentration exist in central cholinergic synapses; astrocytes covering these synapses are able to synthesize and release the acetylcholine binding protein (AChBP), which structurally is similar to the nicotinic cholinoreceptor and has a high-affinity binding site for ACh. Extensive stimulation of cholinergic terminals enhances the release of AChBP, which enters the synaptic cleft, binds ACh and effectively lowers the concentration of the latter, thus attenuating the synaptic strength.

Second, 'glio' transmitters released from astrocytes also affect synaptic transmission in neighbouring neuronal circuits. In fact, astrocytes are capable of exerting multiple effects on this ongoing neurotransmission. For example, in hippocampal neurones cultured together with astrocytes, the stimulation of the latter increased the frequency of spontaneous (miniature) excitatory and inhibitory postsynaptic currents, but decreased the amplitude of the evoked postsynaptic responses (Figure 7.13). This difference was explained through activation of two independent pathways: in the former case, glutamate acted via presynaptic NMDA receptors (which are active already at low glutamate concentrations), whereas the latter effect was mediated through presynaptic metabotropic glutamate receptors. Astroglial glutamate release may also affect inhibitory pathways in the hippocampus, by facilitating GABA release from interneurones connected to pyramidal CA1 cells; this effect is mediated by activation of ionotropic glutamate receptors of the kainate subtype, located in the terminals of the interneurones.

Astrocytes are also capable of modulating synaptic transmission through the release of ATP. In hippocampal neuronal–glial co-cultures, ATP secreted by astrocytes inhibited glutamatergic synapses via presynaptic metabotropic (P2Y) purinoreceptors. Alternatively, as was shown in experiments in hippocampal slices, ATP released by astrocytes was catalyzed by ectoenzymes into adenosine, which produced tonic suppression of synaptic transmission by acting on adenosine receptors. Similar effects have been observed in the retina, where ATP released from Müller cells degrades to adenosine and inhibits neurones acting through adenosine receptors.

7.11.1   Morphological plasticity of astroglial synaptic compartment

Astrocytes are able to directly influence synaptic transmission in certain brain regions by changing their morphology and thus remodelling the structure of the

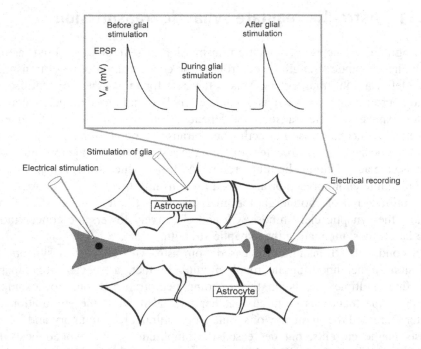

Figure 7.13 Example of modulation of synaptic transmission by glia. Stimulation of astrocytes in astroglial neuronal co-cultures significantly reduces the amplitudes of glutamatergic excitatory postsynaptic potentials (EPSPs) in neighbouring neurones. (Modified from Araque A, Parpura V, Sanzgiri RP Haydon PG (1998) Glutamate-dependent astrocyte modulation of synaptic transmission between cultured hippocampal neurons. *Eur J Neurosci* **10**, 2129–2142)

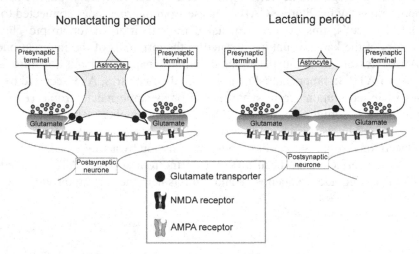

Figure 7.14 Morphological plasticity of astroglia in hypothalamus. Upon lactation astrocyte processes shrink, thus allowing more glutamate in the synaptic cleft, thereby strengthening synaptic transmission. (Modified from Sykova E (2004) Extrasynaptic volume transmission and diffusion parameters of the extracellular space *Neuroscience* **129**, 861–876)

synapse. The most prominent example of such morphological plasticity is observed in the supra-optic nucleus. During lactation (which is associated with high levels of oxytocin), astrocytes withdraw their processes from synapses, which increases the effective extracellular glutamate concentration and decreases glutamate uptake, thereby strengthening glutamatergic transmission (Figure 7.14).

7.12   Integration in neuronal–glial networks

The two types of intercellular signalling – wiring transmission and volume transmission – are involved in information transfer in neuronal–glial networks. Neurones and glia are integrated in many ways, which involve homocellular and heterocellular contacts (Figure 7.15). Homocellular contacts are represented by neuronal–neuronal chemical synapses and electrical synapses formed by gap junctions between neurones and between glial cells (wiring transmission). Heterocellular contacts between neurones and glia are formed by either direct synapses formed by neuronal terminals on glial cells (wiring transmission; and, at least in the case of NG2-glia, direct synapses formed by NG2-glial processes on neurones), or by close apposition of neuronal terminals and perisynaptic astroglial processes. In the latter case, neurotransmitter released by neurones activates astrocyte membranes by spillover from the synaptic cleft (volume transmission). Astroglial cells signal back to neurones through the release of neurotransmitters (either vesicular or transplasmalemmal), which may activate several neurones simultaneously by the way of volume transmission. At the same time, neurotransmitters released by astrocytes may signal homocellularly and, together with astroglial–astroglial gap junctional contacts, trigger propagating calcium waves within the glial syncytium. Astrocyte–neuronal signalling may operate either locally, by feeding back to the active synaptic domain, or distantly; in the latter case the astroglial Ca^{2+} wave stimulated by synaptic activation conveys the signal through the astroglial network and initiates transmitter release distantly, to affect neurones not connected synaptically to the primary loci of stimulation.

7.13   Astrocytes as cellular substrate of memory and consciousness?

Contemporary neuroscience regards neuronal networks, and neuronal networks only, as the substrate of memory and consciousness. More than that, current understanding, in essence, denies the existence of special cells or cellular groups which can be the residence of memory, consciousness and other high cognitive functions. At the same time, information processing in the neuronal networks relies entirely on a simple binary code, which might not necessarily offer sophistication sufficient enough to explain how the human brain thinks and becomes

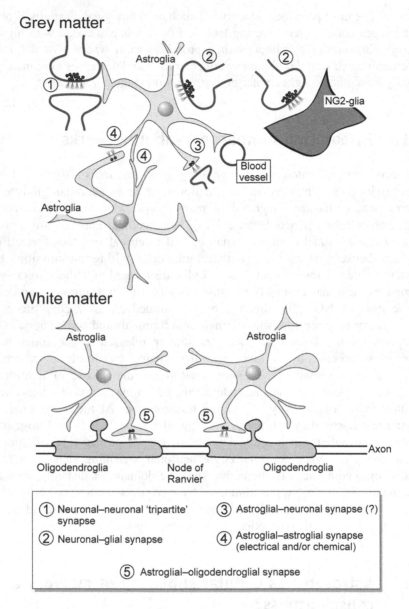

Figure 7.15 Diversity of synaptic contacts between neural cells. In the grey matter, synapses may include: (1) classic 'tripartite' neuronal–neuronal contacts, enwrapped by astroglial membranes; (2) neurone–glial synapses (which have already been discovered for neurone–astroglial and neurone–NG2-glial cell contacts); (3) astroglial–neuronal synapses (which are yet to be discovered); and (4) astroglial–astroglial synapses, which may exist as electrical/gap junctional or chemical contacts. In the white matter, astrocytes may act as presynaptic elements in astroglial–oligodendroglial synapses (5); astrocytes and NG2-glia also contact nodes of Ranvier and so could potentially form synapses with axons at nodes of Ranvier. (Modified from Verkhratsky A, Kirchhoff F (2007) NMDA receptors in glia *Neuroscientist* **13**, 1–10)

self-aware. In contrast, the astroglial syncytium allows much more diverse routes for informational exchange (as intracellular volume transmission allows passage of many important molecules within the connected astroglial network). Astrocytes divide the space of the grey matter into individual domains, where all neuronal and nonneuronal elements are controlled by a single astroglial cell. By extensive contacts with synaptic membranes belonging to these domains, every astrocyte can integrate all the information flowing though neuronal networks, and is capable of regulating these neuronal networks through the release of neurotransmitters, regulation of the extracellular environment and by affecting neuronal metabolism. The individual microdomains are further integrated through intercellular contacts, which multiply the processing capabilities. As a result, it is entirely possible (and conceptually simpler) to conceive how astrocytes may provide the substrate for memory and cognition, whereas neurones are specialized to serve as the transducers of information between different brain regions and between the brain and the rest of the body. Will such an 'astrocentric' theory stand the scrutiny of experimental testing? This has to be seen in the future.

8

Oligodendrocytes, Schwann Cells and Myelination

The function of oligodendrocytes is to produce the myelin sheaths that insulate axons in the CNS. Myelinating Schwann cells serve the same function in the PNS, but there are also significant populations of nonmyelinating and perisynaptic (terminal) Schwann cells (Figure 8.1). Myelinating and nonmyelinating Schwann cells are equally numerous. These multiple Schwann cell types perform many of the diverse functions performed by astrocytes in the CNS – such as structure, metabolism, regulation of the microenvironment, and signalling. These functions are absolutely vital for PNS development, physiology and pathology. In contrast, oligodendrocytes can be defined by their exclusive function of myelination. There are 'nonmyelinating oligodendrocytes' in the CNS grey matter, but they are minor populations and their functions are unknown; it is even questioned that they are oligodendrocytes.

Myelinating Schwann cells or oligodendrocytes and the axons they support are interdependent functional units. The development of myelinating cells depends on a series of coordinated signals from axons. Similarly, the radial growth of axons (axon's diameter) and the myelin sheath (number of lamellae) are interdependent, resulting in the g-ratio of axons: number of myelin lamellae (1:10), which is a constant in the CNS and PNS. Furthermore, mature axons and myelinating cells continue to depend on each other for normal function and integrity: the loss of axons results in degeneration of oligodendrocytes and de-differentiation of Schwann cells; conversely, axons degenerate in the absence of appropriate support from Schwann cells and oligodendrocytes. The relationship between myelinating cells and axons is perhaps the clearest demonstration of the interdependence of neurones and glia.

Nonmyelinating Schwann cells surround bundles of small-diameter unmyelinated axons. These serve multiple functions, physically supporting and separating unmyelinated axons with fine processes, as well as providing physiological support in the form of ion homeostasis and preventing ephaptic transmission between axons. Mature nonmyelinating Schwann cells express a number of surface

Glial Neurobiology: A Textbook   Alexei Verkhratsky and Arthur Butt
© 2007 John Wiley & Sons, Ltd   ISBN 978-0-470-01564-3 (HB); 978-0-470-51740-6 (PB)

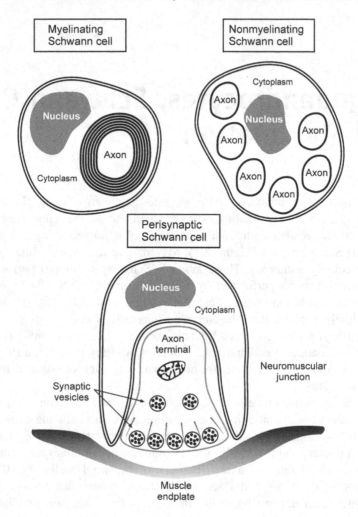

Figure 8.1 Schwann cells. There are equal numbers of myelinating and nonmyelinating Schwann cells in the PNS. *Myelinating Schwann cells* myelinate a single axon, which has a critical diameter above 1 μm. *Nonmyelinating Schwann cells* ensheath multiple unmyelinated axons, which are smaller than the critical diameter of 1 μm. *Perisynaptic (terminal) Schwann cells* ensheath terminal axonal branches and synaptic boutons at the neuromuscular junction; their basal lamina fuses with that of the muscle fibre and motor endplate

molecules characteristic of immature Schwann cells that are not found on mature myelinating Schwann cells, including the cell adhesion molecule L1 and neural cell adhesion molecule (NCAM). In addition, nonmyelinating Schwann cells can adopt a myelinating phenotype under experimental conditions.

Perisynaptic (terminal) Schwann cells at the neuromuscular junction (NMJ) ensheath terminal axonal branches and synaptic boutons. They are covered by a basal lamina that fuses with that of the muscle fibre and motor endplate.

Perisynaptic Schwann cells play essential roles in synaptic function, maintenance, and development. In addition, they respond to nerve activity by increased intracellular Ca^{2+} and are capable of modulating synaptic function in response to pharmacological manipulations. During development they contribute to the maturation and extension of the motor endplate and they stabilize the NMJ. They also regulate the efficacy of synaptic transmission and neurotransmitter release by modulating perisynaptic ions and Ca^{2+} concentration, and may also induce postsynaptic acetylcholine receptor aggregation. Furthermore, in regeneration perisynaptic Schwann cells guide the growth of regenerating presynaptic nerve terminals at adult NMJs.

Schwann cell basal lamina. A major difference between Schwann cells and oligodendrocytes is that Schwann cells form a basal lamina around their abaxonal cytoplasmic membranes. In longitudinal section, the basal lamina forms a continuous tube along the axon, bridging the nodal gap between Schwann cells. In contrast, oligodendrocytes and CNS myelin do not have a basal lamina, and myelin sheaths are directly apposed to each other within bundles or fascicles. The major constituents of the basal lamina are the extracellular matrix (ECM) components, laminin-2 (merosin), heparan sulphate proteoglycans (e.g. perlecan, agrin), collagen type IV, and fibronectin. The basal lamina is crucial for myelination, and its disruption results in severe dysmyelination, as for example in dystrophic mice which lack laminin-2. Schwann cells express a number of receptors for basal lamina components, including dystroglycan-dystrophin-related protein 2 (DRP2) and integrins (e.g. $\alpha6/\beta1$), which are essential for myelination. In addition, many of the ECM components of the basal lamina promote axon growth and are therefore important during PNS regeneration.

8.1 The myelin sheath

The myelin sheath is a fatty insulating layer that facilitates saltatory conduction of action potentials. Myelin sheaths serve the same function as the plastic insulating coating around electrical wires. However, unlike plastic coating, myelin is a living material that has to be continuously produced throughout life by highly specialized myelinating cells – oligodendrocytes in the CNS and Schwann cells in the PNS.

8.1.1 Myelin structure

The myelin sheath is wrapped around the axon to form concentric layers or *lamellae*, which are best seen in transverse section (Figure 8.2). Longitudinally along axons, consecutive myelin sheaths are separated by *nodes of Ranvier*, the highly specialized areas of naked axonal membrane where action potentials are propagated (see Chapter 8.4). The myelin sheath between nodes is therefore called

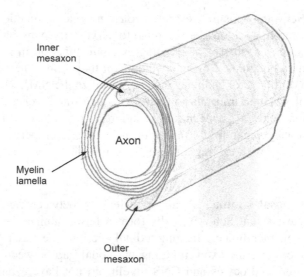

Figure 8.2 The myelin sheath in transverse section. The myelin sheath is seen to be formed by multiple layers of compacted *myelin lamellae* that spiral around the axon. The *inner mesaxon* and *outer mesaxon* are cytoplasmic ridges which pass along the length of the myelin sheaths, and are contiguous with the cell body (see Figure 8.4). This basic structure of the myelin sheath is the same in both PNS and CNS

the internode. Complex axo–glial junctions between the terminal ends of the myelin sheath (*paranodal loops*) and the axolemma at *the paranode* are important in the separation of Na^+ and K^+ channels that are respectively clustered at the node of Ranvier and under the myelin sheath in *the juxtaparanode*. A major difference between PNS and CNS nodes is that myelinating Schwann cells extend microvilli to fill the nodal gap, whereas oligodendrocytes do not have microvilli and the function of providing perinodal processes is fulfilled by astrocytes and NG2-glia (Figure 8.3). Perinodal processes play an important role in stabilizing axo–glial interactions at the node and in ion homeostasis. In addition, the PNS node is completely covered by the basal lamina, which is absent in the CNS.

Myelin is one of the most complex cellular structures in the brain. If unwrapped, the myelin sheath would appear as an extraordinarily large trapezoid or spade-like extension of the glial cell plasmalemma; a single sheet in Schwann cells (Figure 8.4) and multiple sheets in oligodendrocytes (Figure 8.5). The myelin sheets are continuations of the cell membrane, in which most of the cytoplasm is extruded so that the apposing phospholipid bilayers are fused to form the lamellae of *compacted myelin*. The fusion of apposed cytoplasmic interfaces of the plasma membrane forms the *major dense line* of the myelin sheath, whilst fusion of the outer interfaces of the plasma membrane forms the minor dense line or *intraperiod line*, as seen in transverse section under the electron microscope (Figure 8.6). There is a ridge of cytoplasm around the edge of the compacted myelin sheath and isolated strands of cytoplasm within the compacted myelin – called

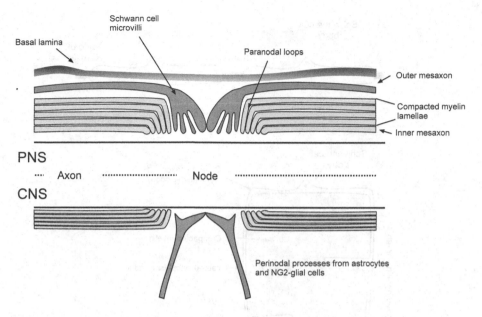

Figure 8.3 The myelin sheath in longitudinal section. Myelin sheaths are separated along the length of axons by nodes of Ranvier, the sites of axonal action potential propagation. The myelin sheath between two nodes comprises the compacted *internodal* myelin sheath (see Figure 8.2); the internodal axolemma is relatively undifferentiated. The terminals of the internodal myelin sheath form *paranodal loops* ('para' from the Greek for 'alongside'), which are the lateral cytoplasmic ridges of the myelin sheath, stacked one upon the other as the myelin lamellae spiral around the axon (refer to Figures 8.4 and 8.6). The paranodal loops are very tightly apposed to the axolemma, with which they form highly complex junctions. These paranodal axoglial junctions are critical for separating the axolemmal Na^+ (at nodes) and K^+ channels (at *juxtaparanodes*; 'juxta' from the Latin for 'next to'), which are the basis of the action potential (see Figure 8.10). The cytoplasm of the paranodal loops is contiguous with that of the inner and outer mesaxons and the cell body (see Figure 8. 4). These elements are the same in the CNS and PNS. The PNS and CNS differ in that myelinating Schwann cells extend microvilli to fill the nodal gap, and the Schwann cell basal lamina completely covers PNS nodes and internodes to form a tube along the axon. Oligodendrocytes do not form a basal lamina, which is therefore absent from CNS nodes. Neither do oligodendrocytes form microvilli, and this function is performed by the perinodal processes of astrocytes and NG2-glia

Schmidt–Lanterman incisures – which are important for intracellular transport from the cell body to the myelin sheath (see Chapter 8.2.3). When wrapped around the axon, the inner and outer cytoplasmic ridges (or mesaxons) appear to 'corkscrew' around the axon, and the lateral cytoplasmic ridges build up to form the paranodal loops which are apposed to the axolemma by complex axo–glial junctions. Compacted myelin therefore comprises multiple fused phospholipid bilayers and it is these lipids that provide the insulating properties of the sheath. Like other cell membranes, myelin has a high electrical resistance and low capacitance, which is essential for rapid saltatory conduction from node to node.

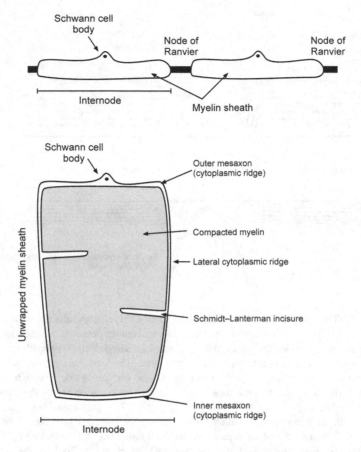

Figure 8.4 Myelinating Schwann cells. There is a 1:1 relationship between a myelinating Schwann cell and the axon it myelinates. Consecutive Schwann cells are separated by *nodes of Ranvier* and the myelin sheaths between nodes are *internodes*; the internodal length is directly related to axon diameter and determines the speed of conduction. Each myelin sheath is a large trapezoid sheet of *compacted myelin* that is wrapped around the axon; the thickness of the myelin sheath determines the insulating properties of the sheath and is directly related to axon diameter (the g-ratio defines the relationship axon diameter (D):the number of myelin lamellae – myelin sheath thickness, which is a constant – 1:10 – in PNS and CNS). Hence, large diameter axons have thicker and longer myelin sheaths (as great as 1000 μm for the largest axons) and conduct action potentials must faster than small diameter axons (see Figure 8.9); this relationship is the same in the PNS and CNS. The sheet of compacted myelin is an extension of the cell plasmalemma (see Figure 8.6), and is completely surrounded by a ridge of cytoplasm. The inner and outer cytoplasmic ridges form the inner and outer mesaxons, respectively (see Figure 8.2), and the lateral ridges form the paranodal loops, which stack upon each other when the sheet of myelin is wrapped around the axon (see Figure 8.3). In the myelin sheaths around larger diameter axons, strands of cytoplasm called *Schmidt–Lantermann incisures* extend into the compacted myelin. The cytoplasm of all these elements is contiguous with that of the cell body and forms the intracellular pathway along which all of the myelin products are transported from the cell body and targeted to the myelin sheath, over hundreds and potentially thousands of microns

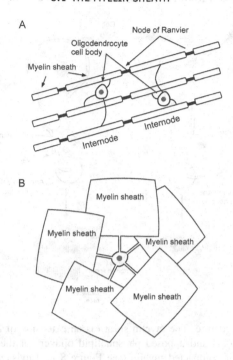

Figure 8.5 Oligodendrocytes:

A. In contrast to Schwann cells, oligodendrocytes myelinate multiple axons. The ratio of oligodendrocyte:axons within the unit varies from 1:1 in type IV oligodendrocytes, 1:5 in type III oligodendrocytes, and 1:30 in type I/II oligodendrocytes. On average, oligodendrocytes myelinate 10 or more axons within approximately 10–30 μm of the cell body; they do not produce consecutive myelin sheaths along the same axon.

B. Each myelin sheath is a large sheet of compacted myelin, with ridges of cytoplasm that are connected to the oligodendrocyte cell body by connecting processes (see Figure 8.4). As in the PNS, there are strict positive relationships between axon diameter and myelin sheath dimensions, and there is also a strict negative relationship between axon diameter and the ratio of oligodendrocyte:axons; type I/II oligodendrocytes myelinate numerous small diameter axons with short, thin myelin sheaths, and type III/IV oligodendrocytes myelinate a small number of large diameter axons with long, thick myelin sheaths. Consequently, there is a sharp demarcation in the volume of myelin supported by type I/II and type III/IV oligodendrocytes, which respectively support myelin volumes of approximately 500 μm³ and 30 000 μm³; oligodendrocytes and Schwann cells that myelinate the largest diameter axons support as much as 150 000 μm³ of myelin

In terms of the volume of plasmalemma supported, oligodendrocytes and Schwann cells are probably the largest cells in the body, with lengths of up to 1 mm. The dimensions of the myelin sheath vary directly with axon diameter: the number of lamellae and internodal length vary approximately from 10–100 and 100–1000 μm, respectively. The volume of myelin supported by an individual cell can be estimated as the internodal length (L) by the width, which is a function of axon circumference (πD), lamellar thickness (d), and the number of times the

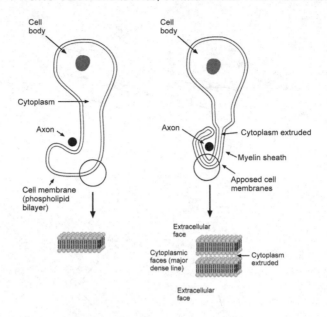

Figure 8.6 Myelin structure. The myelin sheath is an extension of the cell in which most of the cytoplasm is extruded and apposed phospholipid bilayers of the plasmalemma are fused to form the lamellae of compacted myelin (see Figure 8.7). Envisage the myelin sheath as a partly inflated balloon – the air in the balloon represents the cytoplasm, and the rubber of the balloon represents the phospholipid bilayer of the plasmalemma, with inner (cytoplasmic) and outer (extracellular) faces. When the air/cytoplasm is extruded, the balloon deflates and the inner/cytoplasmic faces become apposed. Now, envisage the axon as a pencil, around which the deflated balloon is enwrapped, so that now the outer/extracellular faces become apposed to each other. This is analogous to the structure of the myelin sheath and to the process of myelin compaction. Production and compaction of myelin is a continuous process, whereby myelin components are inserted into the myelin sheath and cytoplasm is extruded. Gap junctions within the myelin sheath play important roles in water and ion transport and myelin compaction in both Schwann cells and oligodendrocytes. Knockout studies indicate a critical role for Cx32 in Schwann cells, whereas this is a function of both Cx32 and Cx47 in oligodendrocytes, in addition to the inward rectifying potassium channel $K_{ir}4.1$. Oligodendrocytes are also rich in the enzyme carbonic anhydrase, which is important in ion and water transport in other tissues (such as the kidney and gut) and may play a similar role in extrusion of cytoplasm from the myelin sheath

sheath is wrapped around the axon, i.e. the number of lamellae (N). Schwann cells have a 1:1 relationship with axons and internodal lengths as great as 1000 μm, so that a cell myelinating a 10–15 μm diameter axon supports a volume of myelin as great as 150 000 μm^3, which would be visible to the naked eye. In oligodendrocytes, there is a sharp demarcation between type I/II oligodendrocyte units, which have a large number of small diameter axons with short, thin myelin sheaths, and type III/IV oligodendrocyte units, which have a small number of axons with long, thick myelin sheaths (see Chapter 3.2). Type I/II oligodendrocytes support approximately 500 μm^3 of myelin, whereas type III/IV oligodendrocytes, like Schwann cells, support $30\,000\text{–}150\,000\,\mu\text{m}^3$ of myelin, depending on axon diameter. The dimensions of the myelin sheath determine the conduction properties of the axons within the unit: the thickness of the myelin sheath determines the insulating properties and the length determines the speed of conduction. Hence, larger axons have longer and thicker myelin sheaths and conduct faster than thinner axons. It should be noted that the myelin sheath is a living structure and its production places a considerable metabolic load on myelinating cells; the turnover of phospholipids and myelin proteins is in the order of days to weeks.

8.1.2 Composition of myelin

The main constituents of myelin are the lipids (70 per cent of its dry weight), the remainder being proteins (30 per cent of its dry weight), which are largely specific to myelin, with subtle differences between PNS and CNS (Figure 8.7). The lipids provide myelin with its insulating properties, whereas the proteins serve to fuse and stabilize myelin lamellae and to mediate membrane–membrane interactions between the myelin lamellae, and between the axon and myelin sheath. Our understanding of their functions comes from studies of their localization and studies in naturally occurring mutations and genetically altered animals.

8.1.2.1 CNS myelin

Lipids *Cholesterol* is a major component of myelin, together with phospholipids and glycolipids, in ratios ranging from 4:3:2 to 4:4:2. Myelin phospholipids are not unusual, but myelin lipids are rich in glycosphingolipids, in particular galactocerebrosides (*GalC*) and their sulphated derivatives, *sulphatides*, which are used immunohistochemically to identify myelinating oligodendrocytes. The functions of GalC have been studied in mice with an inactive gene for the enzyme that catalyzes the final step in the synthesis of GalC (UDP-galactose:ceramide galactosyl transferase (CGT)). These mice have no detectable levels of GalC or sulphatides, and display a pronounced tremor starting at about two weeks (the age after birth when active myelination is at its peak in rodents). The abnormalities of internodal myelin spacing and the complete absence of transverse bands at the paranodal axo–glial junctions indicate an essential role for galactolipids in axon–glial interactions. The role of sulphatides has been examined in mice that lack cerebroside sulphotransferase, which also have disrupted paranodes, as well as greater numbers of differentiated oligodendrocytes.

There are also several minor galactolipids, such as fatty esters of *cerebroside*, and a number of *gangliosides*, GM4 being one of the most abundant in CNS myelin (but only a minor component in PNS), together with LM1 and GM3, which account for the large majority in PNS myelin. Mice lacking complex gangliosides

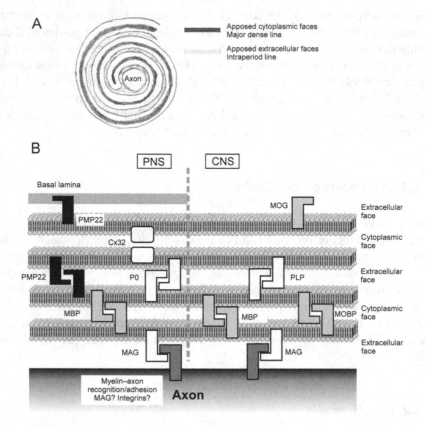

Figure 8.7 Myelin Composition:

A. The myelin sheath comprises layer upon layer of cell membrane and its main constituents are therefore lipids (70 per cent); these give the myelin sheath its insulating properties. The apposed cytoplasmic and extracellular interfaces of the compacted myelin lamellae (see Figure 8.6) respectively form the *major dense line* and *intraperiod line*; their fusion relies on a number of myelin-specific proteins, which are the second major constituents (30 per cent) of the myelin sheath.

B. The compositions of CNS and PNS myelin are largely equivalent, but they differ in a number of specific proteins. In the CNS, the major proteins are MBP and PLP, which respectively fuse the cytoplasmic and extracellular faces of the myelin lamellae; the absence of MBP or PLP respectively results in disruption of the major dense line and intraperiod line of the CNS myelin sheath. PNS myelin also contains MBP and PLP, but their functions are not clear. The major protein in PNS myelin is P0, which makes up more than 50 per cent of PNS myelin and mediates fusion of the myelin lamellae; PMP22 and Cx32 are also essential for PNS myelin formation. MAG is found in both CNS and PNS myelin and is important for membrane–membrane interactions, in particular between the myelin and axon at paranodes; MOG is specific to CNS myelin.

Abbreviations: Cx32, connexin 32; MAG, myelin associated glycoprotein; MBP, myelin basic protein; MOG, myelin oligodendrocyte glycoprotein; P0, protein zero; PLP, proteolipid protein; PMP22, peripheral myelin protein 22

develop both CNS and PNS pathologies characterized by demyelination and axonal degeneration.

Proteins

Myelin proteins are mostly specific to myelin. The major ones are myelin basic protein (*MBP*) and proteolipid protein (*PLP*, and its isoform *DM20*), which constitute about 80 per cent of CNS protein. In addition, there are a number of proteins that make up a small but significant fraction of myelin, including 2′,3′-cyclic nucleotide-3′-phosphodiesterase (*CNP*, 4 per cent), myelin associated glycoprotein (*MAG*, <1 per cent), and myelin oligodendrocyte glycoprotein (*MOG*, <0.1 per cent). Other proteins include myelin/oligodendrocyte specific protein (*MOSP*), myelin-associated/oligodendrocyte basic protein (*MOBP*), oligodendrocyte-myelin glycoprotein (*OMgp*), *Nogo*, *P2*, *transferrin*, *carbonic anhydrase*, and members of the tetraspan-protein family, including oligodendrocyte specific protein (*OSP/claudin-11*), gap junction protein connexins (*Cx32*, *Cx47*), and *tetraspan-2*, together with a number of enzymes that are important for myelin formation and turnover.

MBP is a family of proteins with many isoforms. The main function of MBP appears to be in the fusion of the cytoplasmic interface of the myelin lamellae and formation of the major dense line – a large deletion of the MBP gene in *shiverer* mutant mice results in the loss of the major dense line. Multiple isoforms of MBP are differentially expressed within oligodendrocyte somata and myelin, indicating they have multiple functions.

PLP constitutes up to 50 per cent of CNS myelin proteins, with two isoforms, PLP and DM20. There are spontaneous mutations involving the PLP gene, e.g. the *jimpy* (jp) mouse, myelin deficient (*md*) rats, and the *shaking* pup, and transgenic knockout mice have been developed. These studies indicate that PLP is important for fusing the extracellular face of the myelin lamellae and forming the intraperiod line. The absence of PLP/DM20 also results in axonal degeneration. In addition, in *jimpy* mice there are a number of developmental abnormalities, including premature oligodendrocyte cell death.

CNP is specific to oligodendrocytes in the CNS and Schwann cells in the PNS, but the functions of this enzyme in myelin are unresolved. It is expressed early in oligodendrocyte development and is used as a marker for this lineage. There are two isoforms, CNP1 and CNP2. In oligodendrocytes, CNP is localized immunohistochemically to the cell body and processes, rather than compacted myelin. The lack of substrates for this enzyme in myelin has led to the suggestion of alternative functions, such as interaction with the actin cytoskeleton and microtubules to regulate process outgrowth. However, in the Cnp1 knockout mouse, the myelin sheaths appeared normal, although there was axonal degeneration.

MAG is only a minor component of myelin (<1 per cent in the CNS and 0.1 per cent in the PNS), but it is the major glycoprotein. It consists of two isoforms, S(small)- and L(large)-MAG, which are differentially expressed during development. L-MAG is the predominant form in early myelination, but declines during development, and S-MAG is the predominant form in the adult. In the CNS, MAG is confined to the periaxonal cytoplasmic ridges of the myelin sheath, contrasting with a broader distribution in the PNS. MAG function has been studied in MAG knockout mice, where its absence results in abnormal formation of the paranodal loops and periaxonal cytoplasmic ridge, indicating a role for MAG in axon–myelin interactions. MAG is a member of the immunoglobulin (Ig) gene superfamily with significant homology to neural cell adhesion molecule (NCAM). The extracellular domain of MAG possesses the L2/HNK-1 epitope and binds to specific gangliosides on the axon membrane, which participate in recognition and adhesion. The cytoplasmic domain of MAG has several phosphorylation sites, and interacts with several transduction pathways, including *Fyn*, which is essential for myelination, and *S100*β protein, which regulates the cytoskeleton and signal transduction. Hence, MAG is likely to play a major role in signal transduction across the myelin membrane. MAG is also an inhibitor of axon growth, and binds to the same receptor as Nogo and OMgp, with important implications for regeneration in the CNS.

MOG is specific to oligodendrocytes, and is mostly located on the cell surface and outermost lamellae of compacted myelin in the CNS. MOG expression is developmentally regulated and is one of the last myelin proteins to be expressed, making it a marker for mature oligodendrocytes. The function of MOG is unclear, but it is a member of the IgCAM superfamily, and may have similar adhesive and intracellular functions as MAG and P0. CNS myelin does not have a basal lamina and so MOG may be important in adhesion and interactions between adjacent sheaths within axon fascicles. MOG is the main antigen responsible for demyelination in the animal model of demyelination, experimental autoimmune encephalomyelitis (*EAE*).

MOBP is a relatively newly described family of CNS-specific myelin proteins. There are several MOBP isoforms that are relatively abundant and second only to MBPs and PLPs. MOBPs are located in the major dense line, where they may play a similar role to MBP. There are a number of MOBP isoforms that are differentially expressed within oligodendrocyte somata and myelin, suggesting that like MBP they have multiple functions. MOBP knockout mice have not revealed any clear abnormalities in myelin. MOBP has been used to induce EAE in mice and lymphocytes from patients with MS have autoreactivity to MOBP.

P2 is mainly a PNS protein, but is found in human CNS myelin, particularly in the spinal cord.

OMgp   is localized to paranodal areas. Expression appears at the time of myelination and may be important in axon–myelin sheath interactions. OMgp is another component of myelin that inhibits neurite outgrowth by binding to the Nogo receptor. In rat spinal cord, OMgp has been shown to be localized to cells (most likely NG2-glia/synantocytes), whose processes converge to form a ring that completely encircles the nodes. In OMgp knockout mice, nodes were abnormally wide and collateral sprouting was observed, indicating OMgp prevents axonal sprouting.

Nogo-A   is abundantly expressed in both neurones and in oligodendroglial cell bodies and their myelin sheaths. Its function in oligodendrocytes is unresolved, and it is of greatest interest as one of the major axon growth inhibiting proteins in myelin. It is possible that Nogo, with MAG and OMgp, my help restrict axonal growth in the mature CNS.

MOSP   is localized to the extracellular face of myelin, and its function is unresolved. The developmental expression of MOSP at the onset of myelination and the interactions of MOSP with microtubules suggest it may play a role in myelin formation.

Transferrin   (Tf) is an iron transport glycoprotein found throughout the body, but is localized to oligodendrocytes in the CNS and its developmental expression matches myelination. Oligodendrocytes contain the four proteins which are responsible for the regulation and management of iron: transferrin, transferrin receptor, ferritin and iron responsive protein. Iron is a cofactor for several enzymes, and is a basic requirement for oxidative metabolism. Oligodendrocytes contain the highest levels of iron of any cell type in the brain, which may reflect the high metabolic load of myelin production. Studies in transgenic mice overexpressing Tf in oligodendrocytes suggest that Tf stimulates oligodendrocyte differentiation and myelination.

Carbonic anhydrases   (CA) catalyze the reversible hydration of CO_2, and are critical for the H^+ buffering power of the CO_2/HCO_3^- buffer system. Oligodendrocytes may play a significant role in maintaining extracellular and intracellular pH, which is important for ion channel and transmitter receptor function. This is likely to play a role in ion and water movement in the myelin sheath, possibly important in the extrusion of cytoplasm from compacted myelin.

OSP/claudin-11   is structurally similar to *PMP22* found in PNS myelin (see below) and is the third most abundant protein in CNS myelin. Studies of the OSP-deficient mouse indicate it is a *tight junction* protein important for the formation of the parallel arrays of tight junctions within myelin sheaths. In addition, OSP/claudin-11 is important in membrane interactions with the extracellular matrix, modulating proliferation and migration of oligodendrocyte progenitors.

There is also evidence implicating OSP/claudin-11 as an autoantigen in the development of autoimmune demyelinating disease.

Connexins: *Cx32* is expressed by oligodendrocytes but its function is unresolved. Although absence of Cx32 in knockout mice results in peripheral demyelination, CNS myelination is unaffected. *Cx47* expression in the CNS is specific to oligodendrocytes, and is regulated in parallel with myelin genes and partially colocalized with Cx32. Mice lacking either Cx47 or Cx32 are viable, but those lacking both connexins display marked abnormalities in CNS myelin, characterized by thin or absent myelin sheaths, vacuolation, enlarged periaxonal collars, oligodendrocyte cell death, and axonal loss. These studies indicate that gap-junction communication is crucial for CNS myelination, most likely forming a conduit for the movement of ions and water between cytoplasmic (uncompacted) and compacted regions of the myelin sheath.

Tetraspan 2 is expressed by cells of the oligodendrocyte lineage and developmental expression indicates it is likely to play a role in signalling in oligodendrocytes in the early stages of their terminal differentiation into myelin-forming glia and may also function in stabilizing the mature sheath.

8.1.2.2 PNS myelin

The specific galactolipids found in PNS myelin are largely the same as CNS myelin, although some glycolipids such as sulphated glucoronyl paragloboside and its derivatives are specific for PNS myelin. The major CNS myelin proteins are also found in PNS myelin, and the main ones that are special to PNS myelin are peripheral myelin protein zero (*P0*), peripheral myelin protein 22 (*PMP22*), peripheral nerve *P2* protein, and *periaxin*.

P0 is a glycoprotein and a member of the IgCAM superfamily. It constitutes more than 50 per cent of PNS myelin and is highly specific to myelinating Schwann cells, unlike many of the other myelin proteins that are also expressed by oligodendrocytes and nonmyelinating Schwann cells. P0 is the major adhesive and structural element that mediates adhesion of the myelin lamellae, through homotypic interaction between apposing extracellular faces to form the intraperiod line. As such, it serves the same function as PLP in CNS myelin. P0 knockout mice exhibit severe hypomyelination and axon degeneration; initiation of myelination in these mice is normal, but P0 is essential for subsequent differentiation and the spiralling, compaction and maintenance of myelin, and axonal integrity. Mutations in the P0 gene, together with PMP22 and Cx32, are responsible for Charcot-Marie-Tooth neuropathies. Genetic manipulation of these genes has led to the development of animal models of peripheral neuropathies.

P2   is a basic protein and a member of the fatty acid binding protein family, with a high affinity for oleic acid, retinoic acid and retinol. It is expressed on the cytoplasmic side of compacted myelin and may be involved in intracellular fatty acid transport. P2 induces experimental allergic neuritis in animals, used as a model for the PNS demyelinating disease Guillain-Barré syndrome.

PMP22   is a tetraspan membrane glycoprotein that plays an important role in myelin synthesis and assembly. Point mutations in the PMP22 gene, such as those in the *trembler* mouse, result in PNS-specific dysmyelination, with phenotypes comparable to P0 knockout mice. However, development of PMP22 knockout mice showed that total disruption of the PMP22 gene results in hypermyelination and demyelination, indicating that PMP22 regulates the initiation of myelination, myelin sheath thickness, and the stability of myelin. In addition, studies in PMP22 knockout mice indicate that PMP22 is a binding partner in the integrin/laminin complex and is involved in mediating the interaction of Schwann cells with the basal lamina.

MBP   is present but it may not play a major role in myelin compaction, and its function may be interchangeable with P0. In *shiverer* mice, the loss of MBP results in severe hypomyelination in the CNS, but PNS myelin appears normal.

PLP/DM20   is found in Schwann cells and PNS myelin, but its function is unclear. PNS myelin appears normal in PLP knockout mice and most mutations.

MAG   is located in the periaxonal Schwann cell membrane, the internal and external mesaxons, the paranodal loops, and the Schmidt–Lanterman incisures. MAG has the same function in PNS and CNS myelin, participating in axonal recognition, adhesion and maintenance of myelin integrity.

Cx32   is found mainly in the paranodal regions and Schmidt–Lanterman incisures. Cx32 is supposed to form gap junctions within the myelin sheath, as well as between Schwann cells, and to be important for ion homeostasis. In addition, Cx32 gap junctions link the partially compacted second layer of myelin to the noncompact outer tongue. The presence of mutations in the X-linked Cx32 gene in Charcot-Marie-Tooth disease type X indicates a role for Cx32 in formation and maintenance of PNS myelin. Cx32 knockout mice have a similar phenotype and develop late-onset demyelination.

Periaxin   is a PNS-specific glycoprotein representing about five per cent of total myelin protein. There are two isoforms, S- and L-periaxin. L-periaxin is a constituent of the DRP2 complex linking the Schwann cell cytoskeleton to the basal lamina. The expression of periaxin is developmentally regulated, being first concentrated in the adaxonal membrane as Schwann cells first ensheath axons, but becoming predominately localized to the abaxonal Schwann cell membrane

apposing the basal lamina as myelin sheaths mature. The shift in localization suggests that periaxin participates in membrane-protein interactions that are
required to stabilize the mature myelin sheath. Mutations in the periaxin gene
cause autosomal recessive Dejerine–Sottas neuropathy and severe demyelinating
Charcot-Marie-Tooth disease. Periaxin knockout mice myelinate normally, but
develop a demyelinating peripheral neuropathy.

8.1.3 Intracellular transport of myelin components

The formation of the myelin sheath is a highly complex process that involves a
number of steps, from mRNA transcription to protein translation and assembly
into the membranes. All of the myelin products have to be transported from the
cell body and targeted to the 'workface' of the myelin sheath, over hundreds and
potentially thousands of microns via the connecting branches (in oligodendrocytes), and along the outer cytoplasmic ridge, down the paranodal loops, into the
inner cytoplasmic ridge and Schmidt–Lanterman incisures. Lipids are probably
targeted to the myelin sheath by associations with proteins, and *lipid rafts* provide
a mechanism by which lipids and proteins are delivered to growing membrane.
However, movement over hundreds of microns is achieved by intracellular transport involving microtubules and other components of the cytoskeleton, which
are similar in oligodendrocytes and Schwann cells. One of the most interesting
aspects of protein targeting in myelinating cells is the phenomenon of MBP mRNA
translocation from the cell body to the myelin sheaths. The MBPs are highly
cationic polypeptides that interact with virtually any negatively charged molecule.
Consequently, MBP is not translated in the cell body, where its interactions with
other cellular components would impede its transport to the myelin sheath. Instead,
the MBP mRNA is translocated in ribonucleoprotein granules along microtubules
to the distal cytoplasmic ridges of the myelin sheath, where the protein is translated 'on site'. PLP and the other main proteins are translated within the cell
body and the protein is transported to the distal myelin sheath. Hence, *in situ*
hybridization clearly shows MBP mRNA in the cell body, processes and myelin
sheaths of oligodendrocytes, whereas PLP mRNA is localized to the cell body.
In contrast, immunostaining for the proteins shows MBP localized within the
myelin sheath and PLP within the cell body, processes and myelin sheath. In
all cases, transport is along microtubules. Translocated MBP mRNA contains an
A2RE element that binds the hnRNP A2 protein, and the mRNA granule-hnRNP
A2 protein complex is transported along microtubules in the processes, dependent
on the microtubule associated protein (MAP) TOG2. The two major MAPs in
oligodendrocytes, MAP2 and tau, regulate microtubule assembly and are critical
for oligodendrocyte differentiation and myelination. The importance of microtubules is demonstrated in the *taiep* rat, where microtubular dysfunction results
in the accumulation of MBP mRNA and myelin proteins in the cell bodies and
dysmyelination. In addition, oligodendrocytes are disrupted in familial multiple

system tauopathy, and oligodendroglial degeneration is the histological hallmark of multiple system atrophy (MSA).

Other components of the cytoskeleton are also essential for process outgrowth and myelin formation. Disruption of the actin cytoskeleton prevents spiralling of the myelinating process in Schwann cells. Rho kinase (ROCK) is a key regulator of myelinating process extension in Schwann cells and oligodendrocytes. ROCK phosphorylates myosin and is an effector of Rho, which regulates the actin cytoskeleton. ROCK signalling regulates the 1:1 relationship between Schwann cells and axons, and disruption of ROCK results in Schwann cells myelinating multiple internodes. In oligodendrocytes, activation of ROCK results in myelin process retraction involving S1P5 and Fyn. By contrast, activation of Cdc42 by Fyn causes process extension.

8.2 Myelination

8.2.1 Functional development of oligodendrocytes

During development, both oligodendrocytes and Schwann cells pass through a number of physiologically distinct stages that can be identified by the expression of stage-specific antigens and are characterized by marked changes in proliferation, migration, morphology and function. Oligodendrocyte progenitor cells (OPCs) develop in highly localized ventricular zones in the brain and spinal cord, by a process that depends on the transcription factors Olig1, Olig2, SOX10 and Nkx2.2, and the signalling molecules sonic hedgehog (Shh), bone morphogenic protein (BMP), and Notch. These transcription factors regulate key stages of OPC development and oligodendrocyte specification; Olig2 and Nkx2.2 are expressed by NG2-glia and have a continued role in the generation of oligodendrocytes throughout life. OPC migrate to their final sites in the brain and spinal cord, where they undergo local proliferation and differentiation, or apoptosis, in response to diffusible growth factors, interactions with the extracellular matrix, and diffusible and membrane-bound signals from axons and glia. OPCs can be identified by their expression of platelet-derived growth factor alpha receptors (PDGFαR), the GD3 ganglioside, and the NG2 CSPG. As OPCs differentiate they gain expression of the sulphatides recognized by the O4 antibody and develop into cells variously called pro-oligodendrocytes, pre-oligodendrocytes, or promyelinating oligodendrocytes. These 'promyelinating' oligodendrocytes lose PDGFαR, GD3 and NG2 as they gain expression of GalC, without losing O4. As these cells form contacts with their target axons they exit the cell cycle and develop into premyelinating oligodendrocytes, which begin to express myelin-related gene products, prior to axon ensheathment and myelination. CNP is one of the earliest oligodendrocyte-specific proteins expressed, and the two isoforms are temporally regulated, with CNP2 being expressed by OPCs, and both CNP1 and CNP2 being expressed at the time of oligodendrocyte differentiation. This is followed by expression of MBP, PLP and

MAG, prior to myelination. The antibody Rip is a useful tool for studying terminal oligodendrocyte differentiation and myelination, but its epitope is unknown. The expression of PLP/DM20 is of interest, because DM20 dominates during the early stages of development and the mRNA can be expressed by OPCs. During differentiation, DM20 declines and PLP is the dominant form during myelination and later. MOBPs are expressed in the late stages of myelination, significantly later than expression of MBP. MOG is one of the last myelin proteins to be expressed and is often used as a marker for mature oligodendrocytes.

The various markers determine oligodendrocyte functions at different stages of differentiation. PDGFαR mediates the effects of PDGF-AA, which is a potent mitogen and survival factor for OPCs and stimulates migration. The loss of PDGFαR signifies a decrease in the migratory and proliferative capacity of OPCs, and a switch to the dependence on axon-derived factors for survival and differentiation. The precise functions of GD3 and NG2 in OPCs are unresolved, but their interactions with the ECM, integrins and the intracellular cytoskeleton indicate they are likely to mediate migration, process outgrowth, cell–cell recognition and adhesion. The developmental expression of galactolipids, sulphatides and myelin proteins are essential for myelination and axon development and integrity. The early expression of CNP, PLP and MAG are likely to be important in process outgrowth, axon recognition, and ensheathment (see Chapter 8.3.3).

Oligodendrocyte differentiation is regulated by a variety of growth factors. PDGF-AA is the best characterized mitogen and survival factor for OPCs. Fibroblast growth factor 2 (FGF2) is a mitogen for OPCs and inhibits their differentiation into oligodendrocytes, at least partly by maintaining expression of PDGFαR. Expression of FGF receptors is developmentally regulated in oligodendrocytes: FGF-R1 increases as cells mature; FGF-R2 is expressed throughout the lineage; FGF-R3 is expressed transiently by premyelinating oligodendrocytes and is important in the initiation of myelination. Insulin-like growth factor I (IGF-I) is a survival factor for oligodendrocytes and with thyroid hormone promotes differentiation. The precise interactions of these trophic factors *in vivo* are unresolved. When OPCs reach their final destinations, contact with axons may be sufficient for survival and differentiation, under the influence of neuregulin-1 (NRG-1) and Notch/Jagged signalling.

8.2.2 Functional development of Schwann cells

Schwann cell precursors originate from neural crest cells that migrate from the dorsal part of the neural tube as it closes. These cells are multipotent and give rise to both neurones and Schwann cells in the PNS. Under the influence of Delta/Notch signalling, NRG-1 and the transcription factor SOX10, crest cells develop first into Schwann cell precursors and then immature Schwann cells. These then diverge to form either nonmyelinating Schwann cells which surround small diameter axons, or myelinating Schwann cells which surround and subsequently myelinate large diameter axons, under the influence of the transcription factor Krox-20 and axonal signals, a key one being NRG-1. NRG-1 is involved in all stages of Schwann cell development, and is the major axon-derived mitogen, survival factor and regulator of myelination for Schwann cells.

8.2.3 Axon–glial interactions and the control of myelination

The ensheathment and myelination of axons during development proceeds in a series of steps that requires complex and reciprocal interactions between axons and the myelinating cells (Figure 8.8). In the first phase, oligodendrocytes and Schwann cells have to recognize axons that require myelination. In a second phase, the processes of the premyelinating cell must adhere to the axons and begin to ensheath them. In a third phase, axons and the myelinating cells pass through a series of interdependent maturation stages. How do the myelinating cells recognize axons to be myelinated? What determines the longitudinal and radial growth of the myelin sheath? How do the myelinating cells regulate the radial growth of axons and what are the signals that determine the differential and highly specialized organization of the axolemma and myelin sheaths at nodes of Ranvier, paranodes, and juxtaparanodes? We do not know the answers to these questions, but there is clear evidence of crucial roles for a number of candidate molecular cues and signals. The answers to these questions will also be relevant to the regulation of remyelination in demyelinating diseases and following regeneration.

Phase 1 – Axon contact: Axon diameter is a critical determinant of myelination in the PNS, and axons are not myelinated until they attain a *critical diameter* of approximately 0.7 μm. Axon diameter plays a less definitive role in the CNS, but nonetheless CNS axons are not myelinated below 0.2 μm and the initiation of myelination only occurs when axons have reached this 'critical' diameter. How the myelinating cells recognize axons of a critical diameter is not yet resolved, but the axonal surface proteins NCAM and L1 are key candidates for negative and positive recognition signals. Disappearance of NCAM from the axonal surface is coincident with the onset of myelination, and suppression of NCAM stimulates myelination. Thus, myelinating cells may distinguish axons that are, and are not, ready for myelination by their differential expression of NCAM. L1 is another adhesion molecule expressed at the axon surface and has a demonstrated function in axon recognition in the PNS and most likely functions in the same way in the CNS. L1 is expressed by premyelinated axons and is down-regulated during myelination. Disruption of L1 strongly inhibits myelination, suggesting an inductive role for L1 in the initiation of myelination (although the L1 knockout mouse shows no abnormalities in myelination). The binding partners for NCAM and L1 in oligodendrocytes have not been identified. In Schwann cells, integrins and periaxin are important in axo–glial interactions. Oligodendrocytes do not express periaxin,

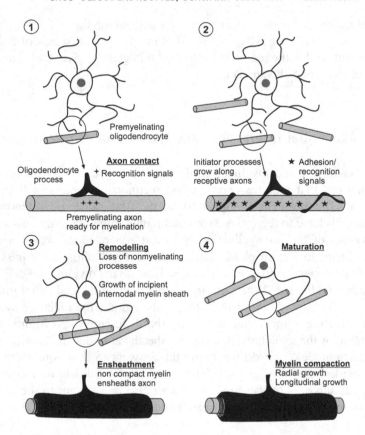

Figure 8.8 Myelination. During development, myelination proceeds in a series of steps that require complex and reciprocal interactions between axons and the myelinating cells (an oligodendrocyte is illustrated). In essence, these interactions are the same in the PNS and CNS, although specific signals regulating myelination may differ; a major difference is that Schwann cells identify a single axon which they myelinate, whereas oligodendrocytes identify multiple axons that require myelination and the definitive number depends on oligodendrocyte phenotype and axon diameter. *Phase 1* – the premyelinating Schwann cell or oligodendrocyte contacts many premyelinated axons, but only those that have attained a critical diameter are myelinated; the recognition and adhesion signals are unresolved, but are likely to involve interactions between membrane surface molecules on the myelinating cell and axon. *Phase 2* – the myelinating cell ensheaths the axon, which requires process adhesion and longitudinal growth; the adhesion molecules have not been identified, although cell surface molecules are again likely candidates, and include MAG and NCAM. At this stage, oligodendrocytes undergo remodelling, when nonensheathing processes are lost and the definitive number of sheaths per unit is established; this is strictly dependent on the diameter of axons in the unit, but the signals controlling oligodendrocyte phenotype (I–IV) divergence are unresolved. *Phases 3 and 4* – axons and the myelin sheath undergo interdependent growth and maturation. Myelin sheaths become compacted and the number of lamellae increases as the axons grow in diameter. Nodes of Ranvier are established (see Figure 8.11) and internodal myelin sheaths grow in direct relationship to the thickening of axons. The longitudinal and radial growth of the myelin sheath and axons, and the organization of the axolemma and myelin sheaths at nodes of Ranvier, paranodes, and juxtaparanodes must involve highly complex molecular cues and signals (see the text for more details)

but specific integrins expressed on oligodendrocytes promote either differentiation and/or proliferation, dependent on the Src family kinases (SFKs) Fyn and Lyn. Early in the lineage, Lyn drives integrin-dependent progenitor proliferation, whereas at later stages Fyn regulates integrin-driven myelin formation and switches the response to neuregulin signalling from proliferation to differentiation. There is experimental evidence that N-cadherin may be important for the initial contact between myelinating oligodendrocytes and axons. Oligodendrocytes also express neurofascin, which is a ligand for the axonal L1 CAM family, but these interactions are likely to play a later role in myelination rather than axon contact and recognition.

Contact with axons stimulates the differentiation of OPCs into premyelinating oligodendrocytes, which begin to sequentially express myelin-related gene products GalC, CNP, PLP/DM20, S-MAG and MBP, prior to axonal ensheathment. Neuregulin-1 and Jagged/Notch signalling are key negative and positive regulators of oligodendrocyte differentiation, respectively. (However, *in vitro* oligodendrocytes will differentiate and form myelin in appropriate culture conditions in the absence of axons.) Down-regulation of axonal Jagged is required for OPC differentiation, and Jagged/Notch signalling may play a particular role in the onset of myelination. Axonal neuregulin-1 induces differentiation of oligodendrocytes *in vitro*. Disruption of neuregulin-1 signalling *in vitro* and the absence of the neuregulin receptor ErbB2 *in vivo* blocks OPC differentiation and myelin formation. In addition, interactions between axonal contactin and Notch receptors on OPCs play an instructive role by promoting OPC differentiation and up-regulation of myelin proteins. In the PNS, NRG-1 type III on axons determines their ensheathment fate, independent of axon diameter, and provides a key instructive signal for Schwann cell myelination.

Phase 2 – Axon ensheathment and establishment of incipient internodal myelin segments: Premyelinating oligodendrocytes that engage axons ready for myelination extend an 'initiator' process that begins to spiral along the axon. The adhesion molecules have not been identified, although MAG and PLP are attractive candidates because of their functions in cell–cell interactions and their timely expression by premyelinating oligodendrocytes. Studies in culture and knockout mice indicate a key role for MAG and NCAM in the initiation of myelination; MAG may increase Fyn tyrosine kinase activity, which is an essential signalling component for oligodendrocyte process outgrowth. Studies in *jimpy* mice indicate that PLP is essential for oligodendrocytes to properly associate with and then ensheath axons. Other signalling molecules such as Tspan-2, neurofascin, and CD9 are abundant in myelinating oligodendrocytes and their processes, and are important for axo–glial interactions, but are probably not essential for the initiation of myelination. Premyelinating oligodendrocytes engage and ensheath multiple axons within 10–30 μm of their cell body. They then go through a remodelling phase, when nonensheathing processes are lost and the definitive number of sheaths per unit is established. The initial lamellar ensheathments are uncompacted (termed

E-sheaths). The clustering of sodium channels at nodes of Ranvier is initiated by these contacts, but functional nodes are established later when incipient internodes have grown (see Chapter 8.4.1). The E-sheaths and presumptive nodes are sufficient to support conduction of axonal action potentials, and they develop concurrently. After the first encirclement of axons, the myelin sheath begins to become compacted (termed M-sheaths) and individual oligodendrocyte units can contain both E- and M-sheaths. The number of axons per oligodendrocyte unit decreases throughout the transition from uncompacted to compacted myelin sheaths. This remodelling occurs in response to unresolved contact-mediated recognition signals derived from axons within the unit, which could be qualitatively and/or quantitatively different for prospective large and small diameter axons. Incipient internodal lengths are also established during the transition to compact myelin, and they have relatively uniform lengths within individual units, subsequently growing symmetrically along the axons to attain their definitive lengths. The longitudinal and radial growth of the myelin sheath is directly dependent on the diameter of axons in the unit. It is not known how myelinated internodal segments become serially arranged along an axon and ultimately attain approximately equal lengths to give rise to the nodal periodicity, which is uniform for any axon of a given diameter. Galactolipids are essential for the internodal myelin spacing, but it seems unlikely they provide the instructive cues.

Phase 3/4 – Remodelling and maturation: After the initial circumnavigation of an axon by a noncompacted sheath, subsequent wraps of the sheath must interact with and fuse to each other, which is dependent on PLP and MBP. The absence of PLP also results in axonal degeneration, indicating a continuing role for PLP in axon–myelin interactions. Longitudinal growth of the myelin sheath is accompanied by maturation of paranodal axo–glial junctions and the maturation of nodes of Ranvier. Knockout studies indicate the development of paranodal axo–glial junctions requires galactolipids, sulphatides, MAG, CNP and connexins. Neurofascin plays a particular role in the establishment of nodes of Ranvier. Maturation of the axon and myelin sheath are interdependent. Radial growth of axons and sodium channel clustering at nodes are dependent on oligodendrocyte and Schwann cell contact. Studies in knockout mice demonstrate that axonal integrity depends on PLP, CNP and GalC. Conversely, loss of axons results in the down-regulation of myelin-related gene products in oligodendrocytes and eventually cell death.

8.2.4 Myelination in the developing PNS

During development, Schwann cells gradually invest smaller and smaller bundles of axons until a 1:1 relationship is established. Schwann cells then undergo substantial elongation along the axon and secrete the basal lamina. The subsequent interactions between the Schwann cell and the basal lamina regulate its differentiation and myelination. Axon diameter is a key factor determining whether an axon is myelinated; every Schwann cell has the potential to myelinate an axon but does so only if it comes into contact with axons with a critical diameter of 0.7 μm. Numerous molecules mediate specific aspects of interactions between Schwann cells and axons. NRG-1 promotes Schwann cell proliferation and survival, and inhibits myelination during development. Before the onset of myelination, Schwann cells express NCAM and L1, both of which play roles in recognition between axons and Schwann cells. L1 on axons and integrins on Schwann cells are essential for ensheathment. On the formation of axon–Schwann cell contact, the expression of NCAM and L1 is down-regulated and MAG is expressed, which mediates the initiation of the myelin spiral. Myelination is accompanied by the expression of P0, which is essential for the spiralling of the myelin sheath and adhesion of the myelin lamellae. Periaxin is important in stabilizing the mature myelin sheath by interactions with the basal lamina. Myelin formation is by the progression of the inner cytoplasmic ridge or lip, which spirals under the compacted myelin (this is opposed to the earlier idea that the Schwann cell itself spiralled around the axon). It is likely that myelin deposition proceeds in the same manner in the CNS, although the picture is complicated by the fact that oligodendrocytes myelinate multiple axons. Longitudinal growth establishes the incipient internodal segment at an early stage, and subsequent growth depends on the developmental lengthening of the nerve. The number of lamellae increases in direct relation to the radial growth of the axon. The two events are interdependent and axons do not attain their adult dimensions in the absence of Schwann cells; increased neurofilament phosphorylation depends on Schwann cell–axon interactions involving MAG.

8.2.5   Electrical activity and myelination

Neural electrical activity has opposing effects on the development of oligodendrocytes and Schwann cells. In the PNS, electrical activity inhibits myelination, by down-regulation of L1 and by the release of ATP to act on P2Y receptors on Schwann cells and inhibit their proliferation, differentiation and myelination. Electrical activity has the opposite effect in the CNS. Blocking (tetrodotoxin) or increasing (alpha-scorpion toxin) neuronal electrical activity respectively inhibit and promote myelination. These effects are mediated by adenosine and ATP released by electrically active axons. Adenosine acts on OPCs, which express A1 receptors, as a potent inhibitor of proliferation, and stimulates their differentiation. ATP acts on astrocytes to trigger them to release leukaemia inhibitory factor (LIF), which in turn acts on oligodendrocytes to promote myelination. The opposing actions of ATP and adenosine on differentiation of Schwann cells and oligodendrocytes provide an explanation for the opposite effects of impulse activity on myelination in the CNS and PNS. In the CNS, glutamate acting on AMPA receptors inhibits OPC proliferation and differentiation, by cell depolarization and blockade of voltage-dependent K^+ channels. It has not been shown whether this is related to neuronal activity.

8.3 Myelin and propagation of the action potential

Creation of the myelin sheath was an extremely important evolutionary step, which dramatically boosted the velocity of nerve impulse propagation, which was critically important for increase in the animal size. The speed of conduction of a given axon is directly and strictly dependent on axon diameter, whereby larger axons conduct faster than smaller diameter axons (Figure 8.9); this is a function of the relationship between the low resistance of the axoplasm and the high resistance and capacitance of the axolemma. The myelin sheath comprises multiple layers of cell membrane (see Chapter 8.8.1), and therefore has ultrahigh resistance and capacitance, enabling smaller diameter axons to conduct impulses much faster than unmyelinated axons of equivalent diameter (Figure 8.9). In nonmyelinated axons the action potential conductance velocity is proportional to half of the axon diameter ($v \propto D/2$), whereas in myelinated ones the speed of impulse propagation is proportional to the axon diameter (Figure 8.9). The maximal nerve impulse conduction velocity, characteristic for thick ($\sim$20–30 μm in diameter) mammalian myelinated axons lies around 80–120 m/s; to achieve the comparable AP propagation speed in nonmyelinated nerves, the axon diameter

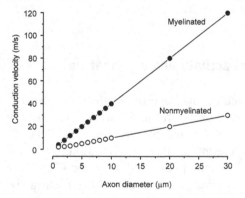

Figure 8.9 Relationship between conduction velocity and axon diameter. Larger axons conduct faster than smaller axons, and the insulation of the myelin sheath enables smaller diameter axons to conduct impulses much faster than unmyelinated axons of equivalent diameter. To achieve the fastest conduction velocities observed in myelinated axons, unmyelinated axons would need to be as large as 500–1000 μm (which is the case in invertebrates). The miniaturization provided by myelin allows the development of highly complex nervous systems seen at their peak in mammals.

(Modified from Waxman SG, Bangalore L (2005) Myelin function and saltatory conduction, In: *Neuroglia*, Kettenmann H & Ransom BR, Eds, OUP, 2005, p. 274)

should be as large as 500–1000 μm. Quite obviously such a thickness would be incompatible with a necessity to pack hundreds of thousands of axons into a single nerve in higher animals. Thus, myelin provides for miniaturization of the nervous system; invertebrates such as the squid, for example, require giant axons (1000 μm diameter) to mediate rapid events such as the contraction of their mantle during the escape reflex. The thinnest myelinated fibres have a diameter ~0.2 μm, and there is very little difference in impulse propagation velocity in nonmyelinated and myelinated fibres at this diameter.

8.3.1 Organization of nodes of Ranvier

The myelin sheath, produced by oligodendrocytes and Schwann cells, divides the axon into myelinated internodal segments, the length of which may vary between 100 μm for small axons to ~1 mm for large-diameter fibres. The internodal segments are separated by nonmyelinated regions, known as nodes of Ranvier (Figure 8.10). The myelin, being a perfect isolator, therefore divides the membrane

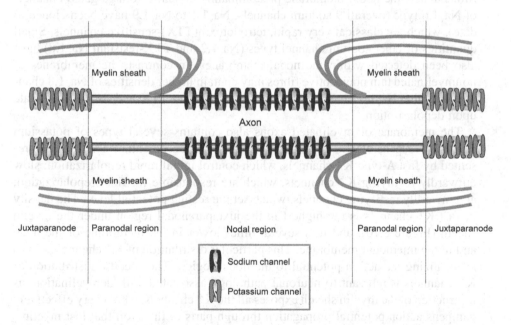

Figure 8.10 The node of Ranvier. Saltatory conduction, whereby action potentials jump from node to node, is dependent on the myelin sheath, because of both its insulating properties and its separation of sodium and potassium channels at nodes of Ranvier. The voltage-gated Na$^+$ channels that generate the upshoot of the action potential are clustered in the nodal axolemma. The voltage-gated K$^+$ channels that are responsible for repolarization of the action potential are localized to the juxtaparanodal region. The complex axoglial junctions between the myelin sheath paranodal loops and axolemma separate the two groups of ion channels, and disruption of these junctions dampens action potential propagation

of nerve fibre into alternating conductive and nonconductive portions. Because of this, the action potential in myelinated axons is shunted from node to node through a low-resistance axoplasm. This propagation is highly reliable (which is achieved by a specific clustering of ion channels, see below) and the safety factor (which is determined as a ratio between the current generated in the node and the current required to stimulate the node) is as big as 5–8. The speed of action potential jumping between the nodes is determined by an internodal conduction time, which at $37\,°C$ is around $20\,\mu s$ (or $0.00002\,s$). The propagation of action potentials through myelinated axons is unidirectional, as the inactivation state of sodium channels (which is induced by depolarization and follows the open state) lasts longer than the internodal conduction time.

The plasma membrane of myelinated axons shows a very specific distribution of voltage-gated channels, which provides a molecular basis for saltatory conduction of action potentials along the nerve fibre. The voltage-gated Na^+ channels, which generate the initial phase of the action potential, are clustered in the nodal membrane at a very high density (>1000 channels/μm^2); in contrast their density in the internodal regions falls sharply to $\sim$20–25 channels per μm^2 (Figure 8.10). Molecularly, the nodal membrane predominantly contains voltage-gated channels of $Na_v1.6$ type (overall 9 sodium channels, $Na_v1.1$ to $Na_v1.9$ have been cloned to date), which are classical very rapid, tetrodotoxin(TTX)-sensitive channels. Small quantities of other sodium channel types ($Na_v1.2$ and TTX-resistant $Na_v1.8$) have also been detected within the nodal membranes. In contrast, the membranes of nonmyelinated thin nociceptive fibres may contain higher densities of $Na_v1.8$ channels and also $Na_v1.9$ channels, which are resistant to TTX and do not inactivate upon depolarization.

The membrane of myelinated axons also contains several types of potassium channels, responsible for repolarization of the action potential. These are represented by fast A-type K^+ channels, which control initial rapid repolarization; slow outwardly rectifying K^+ channels, which are responsible for final repolarization; and inwardly rectifying channels, which set the resting potential level. The density of fast K^+ channels is the highest in the juxtaparanodal region under the myelin sheath (Figure 8.10), and it is several times lower in the membrane of the node and in the internodal membrane. This particular distribution of K^+ channels assists in localizing the action potential to the nodal region. The specific distribution of K^+ channels is relevant to neuronal pathology associated with demyelination, as destruction of the myelin sheath exposes all the K^+ channels, which very effectively dampens action potential propagation through parts of the axon that lost myelin.

Accumulation of voltage-gated sodium channels at the nodes of Ranvier is a prerequisite for saltatory conduction. Clustering is dependent on myelinating Schwann cells and oligodendrocytes, involving the developmental organization of the neighbouring paranodes and juxtaparanodes (Figure 8.11). Molecular components of the nodal, paranodal, and juxtaparanodal zones include cell adhesion molecules and cell-surface molecules involved in cell–cell interactions. The paranodal junction comprises the axon proteins Caspr (paranodin) and contactin,

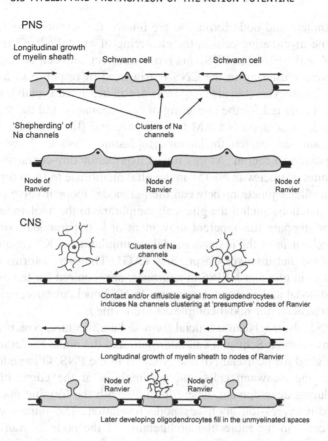

Figure 8.11 Myelinating cells and induction of nodes of Ranvier. Sodium channel clustering at nodes of Ranvier is dependent on the myelinating cells in both the PNS and CNS. Studies during development and following remyelination of demyelinated axons indicate differences between Schwann cells and oligodendrocytes. In the PNS, the clustering of Na^+ channels is dependent on contact by the myelinating Schwann cell; Na^+ channel clusters form at the 'terminals' of the immature myelin sheath and are 'shepherded' along the axolemma as the myelin sheath grows, to combine with consecutive clusters to establish the node of Ranvier. In the CNS, Na^+ channels cluster at presumptive nodes of Ranvier in response to diffusible and contact-mediated signals from oligodendrocytes; subsequently, myelin sheaths grow to 'fill in' the internodal region, and late developing oligodendrocytes fill in any unmyelinated spaces. These models are based on experimental observations, but they leave many questions unanswered. For example, the glia-to-axon and axon-to-glia signals are unknown. Furthermore, it is not clear how the strict relationship between nodal periodicity and axon diameter is established during development; both depend on myelination, but the mechanisms are unknown

and their probable glial partner is neurofascin 155 (NF155). The developmental appearance of these molecules at paranodes coincides with the appearance of constituents of the node, including NF186, ankyrin G, NrCAM and βIV spectrin, closely followed by voltage-gated sodium channels.

Ensheathment and node formation are interrelated events. The first event triggered by the myelinating cells is the clustering of axonal adhesion proteins, such as NrCAM and NF186. In PNS, this requires direct cell–cell contact by Schwann cells, whereas clustering in the CNS is triggered in response to a soluble factor from oligodendrocytes (but also requires contact mediated signals). Recruitment of ankyrin G is required for the clustering of Na^+ channels, and the stability of these clusters is dependent on NrCAM and NF186, and βIV spectrin. As the myelin sheath becomes compacted, the lateral cytoplasmic ridges stack upon each other to form the paranodal region. At this time Caspr/paranodin–contactin complexes in the axolemma interact with NF155 in the glial membrane to form septate-like junctions. Intracellular junctions between the paranodal loops involve connexins. The paranodal junctions anchor the glial cell membrane to the axolemma, and serve as barriers for stopping the apparent movement of juxtaparanodal components. The precise mechanism of the juxtaparanodal accumulation of K^+ channels remains to be determined, but involves Caspr2 and TAG1. The two isoforms of neurofascin (NF), NF155 in glia and NF186 in neurones, are required for the assembly of the specialized nodal and paranodal domains. In NF knockout mice, neither paranodal adhesion junctions nor nodal complexes are formed.

In the PNS, dystroglycan is crucial for nodal architecture, possibly by mediating interactions between Schwann cell microvilli and the nodal axolemma. Gliomedin is a glial ligand for neuronal NF and NrCAM in the PNS. Gliomedin is expressed by myelinating Schwann cells and accumulates at the edges of each myelin segment during development, where it aligns with the forming nodes. Disruption of gliomedin expression abolishes node formation. The impact of myelinating Schwann cells on the molecular architecture of the node of Ranvier is demonstrated in mice deficient in P0. Abnormal myelin formation and compaction results in disruption of nodal sodium channel clustering, with ectopic nodal expression of the $Na_v1.8$ isoform, where it is coexpressed with the ubiquitous $Na_v1.6$ channel. Caspr is distributed asymmetrically or is even absent in the mutant nerve fibres, and the potassium channel $K_v1.2$ and Caspr2 are not confined to juxtaparanodes, but often protrude into the paranodes.

PART III

Glia and Nervous System Pathology

9

General Pathophysiology of Glia

The focus of this book is the normal biology of glia. However, glial cells are involved in almost every type of brain pathology. This is particularly true for microglia, which function primarily in pathology. In this final section of the book, therefore, we introduce some of the important aspects of the role of glia in pathology.

Insults to the nervous system trigger specific reactions of glial cells, generally known as a reactive gliosis, which include the reaction of astroglia (reactive astrogliosis), microglia (activation of microglia) and oligodendroglial and Schwann cells (Wallerian degeneration and demyelination). All these reactions of glial cells are of critical importance for the progress of neural pathology. In the most general terms, one has to remember that astroglial cells can outlive neurones; moreover, the astroglia very often are activated in the presence of dying or already dead neurones; conversely, neurones cannot survive without astrocytes. Similarly, in demyelinating diseases axons cannot function properly when myelinating cells malfunction. Finally, the CNS as a whole has no protection against infection except microglia, and failure of the latter to perform leads to irreparable CNS damage. Beside these, rather profound morphological and biochemical reactions, astroglial cells may be involved in relatively rapid pathological processes, as represented by spreading depression.

9.1 Reactive astrogliosis

All types of brain insults, regardless of aetiology, trigger a complex astroglial response, which is manifested by astrocyte hypertrophy and proliferation. This glial response is defined as *reactive astrogliosis* (Figure 9.1). Reactive astrogliosis is a defensive brain reaction which is aimed at (a) isolation of the damaged area from the rest of the CNS tissue, (b) reconstruction of the blood–brain barrier, and (c) facilitation of the remodelling of brain circuits in areas surrounding the lesioned region. These main tasks are solved in two distinct ways: the reaction of astrocytes close to the insult is very different from that in astroglial cells positioned

Glial Neurobiology: A Textbook   Alexei Verkhratsky and Arthur Butt
© 2007 John Wiley & Sons, Ltd   ISBN 978-0-470-01564-3 (HB); 978-0-470-51740-6 (PB)

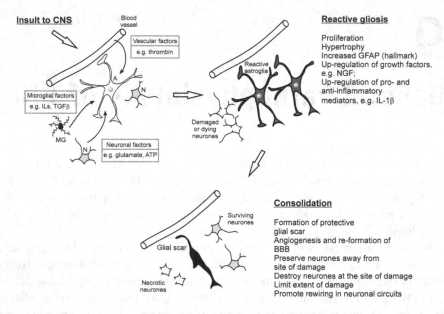

Figure 9.1 Stages of reactive astrogliosis. Insults to the CNS trigger release of numerous factors that interact with astroglial cells and trigger reactive astrogliosis, which is generally represented by hypertrophy and proliferation of astrocytes. Astrogliosis ultimately ends up in complete substitution of previously existing tissue architecture with a permanent *glial scar* (see the text for detailed explanation)

at a distance from the primary lesion. Astrocytes located immediately around the damaged zone undergo a robust hypertrophy and proliferation, which ultimately ends up in complete substitution of previously existing tissue architecture with a permanent *glial scar*; this process is called *anisomorphic* (i.e. changing the morphology) *astrogliosis*. Reactive astrocytes in these areas produce chondroitin and keratin, which inhibit axonal regeneration, and thus prevent nerve processes from entering the damaged zone. Reactive astroglia also release quantities of mucopolysaccharides, which eventually cement the areas of damage, and produce the astrocytic scar.

In astrocytes more distal to the lesion site, the reactive changes are much milder and, although astroglial cells modify their appearance and undergo multiple biochemical and immunological changes, they do not distort the normal architecture of CNS tissue, but rather permit growth of neurites and synaptogenesis, thus facilitating the remodelling of neuronal networks. This type of astrocyte reaction is defined as *isomorphic* (i.e. preserving morphology) *astrogliosis*.

Reactive astrocytes in the areas of isomorphic astrogliosis produce and release several types of growth factors, such as NGF and FGF, and cytokines, such as interleukins. These factors may be important for preservation of neurones from delayed death. Simultaneously, reactive astrocytes synthesize numerous recognition molecules (such as extracellular matrix molecules, cell adhesion molecules, etc.) which promote neuronal–astrocyte interaction and help axonal growth. Therefore, reactive astroglia may either inhibit axonal entry, by forming a nonpermissive scar around the necrotic areas, or assist axonal growth and neuronal remodelling in areas distant to the site of initial insult.

The primary signals, which trigger both forms of astrogliosis, derive from damaged cells in the core of the insult, and are represented by neurotransmitters (most importantly glutamate and ATP), cytokines, adhesion molecules, growth factors, and blood factors (serum, thrombin etc.). The actual combination of these 'damage signals' and their relative concentrations most likely determine the type of astrogliosis experienced by astrocytes in different regions surrounding the initial insult zone.

On a cellular level, insults to the brain, be they ischaemia, trauma or inflammation, result in hypertrophy of astroglial processes and a significant increase in the astrocyte cytoskeleton. The biochemical hallmark of astrogliosis is the upregulation of synthesis of intermediate filament proteins, especially GFAP and vimentin, which together with actin and microtubules form the cytoskeleton. Brain damage very rapidly turns most of the astroglial cells into GFAP-expressing 'reactive' astrocytes. Both GFAP and vimentin are critically important for development of reactive astrogliosis. In animals with genetically deleted GFAP and/or vimentin the astroglial scar is formed slower, it is much less organized and the healing of brain traumas is generally prolonged.

It is still unclear how the normal mature astrocytes are turned into the reactive ones. First, the mature astrocytes can, under the influence of damage-associated signals, dedifferentiate and enter a proliferative state. Alternatively, the reactive astrocytes may arise from astroglial precursors, diffusely dispersed throughout the brain parenchyma, or even from multipotent NG2-expressing precursors and radial glial stem cells. The considerable heterogeneity displayed by reactive astroglial cells most likely indicates that all these routes may be involved in astrogliosis.

9.2 Wallerian degeneration

The severance of axon from the nerve body initiates a series of coordinated events, which produce the disintegration of distal axonal segments, removal of myelin and remodelling of myelinating cells, and finally nerve fibre regeneration, by axonal growth from the nerve slump proximal to the site of insult. This process of nerve degeneration was discovered by Augustus Waller in 1850 and is generally known as 'Wallerian degeneration'.

The term Wallerian degeneration is currently used to describe axonal degeneration in both CNS and PNS; although the properties and underlying processes can be entirely different (Figures 9.2, 9.3). In the PNS, mechanical disruption of the axon triggers demyelination of its distal segment, which begins from the point of the trauma. This demyelination commences within 24–48 hours after the insult and proceeds rather rapidly, with a rate varying between 50 mm/24 hours for the

Wallerian Degeneration in PNS

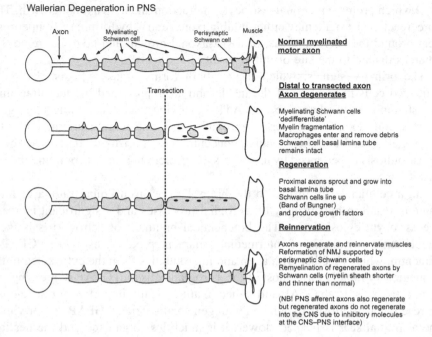

Figure 9.2   General scheme of Wallerian degeneration in the peripheral nervous system

thickest axons to 250 mm/24 hours for the thinnest ones. The process of demyelination goes along with (1), degeneration of the axon, which is soon gone and its
remnants are cleared by phagocytes arriving from neighbouring tissue or blood,
and (2), proliferation of Schwann cells. After complete disappearance of the axon,
the Schwann cells are already prepared to receive the sprouts of growing axons
and begin their myelination. This particular arrangement underlies the remarkable
regeneration potential of PNS (Figure 9.2).

Regeneration of neuromuscular synapses is regulated by perisynaptic Schwann
cells. Following muscle denervation the latter send processes which link the dener-
vated endplates to the regenerating axons.

In the CNS, axonal degeneration after injury proceeds in a different way
(Figure 9.3). First its course is much slower than in the PNS; although the rate
of degeneration depends on phyologenetic and developmental age, being much
faster in the phylogenetically oldest vertebrates (e.g. fish and amphibia) and in
very young mammals. Second, there is no specific reaction from the myelinating
cells: after the myelin sheath of the degenerating axon disintegrates, the nearby
oligodendrocytes do not show any signs of plastic changes or proliferation. In addition, activation of microglia and invading macrophages is incomplete compared
to peripherally, and myelin debris is not effectively removed. Furthermore, reactive astrocytes and NG2-glia migrate to the site of axonal damage and replace

Wallerian Degeneration in CNS

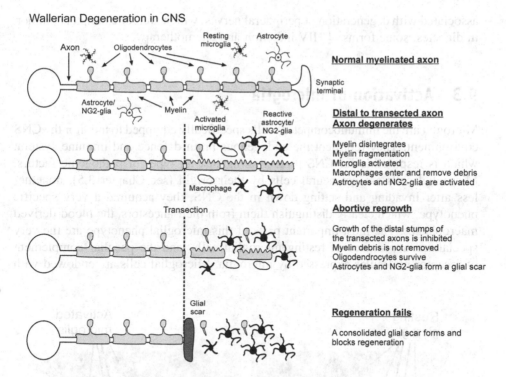

Figure 9.3 General scheme of Wallerian degeneration in the central nervous system

the remnants of the nerve fibres with the astroglial scar. These determine the regeneration failure in damaged CNS axonal fibres.

For many years, axonal degeneration following intersection was regarded as a result of ceased support form the cell body. Recently it became obvious, however, that Wallerian degeneration in the PNS is a specialized active process, which is not very dependent on the links with neuronal somata, but rather involves activation of localized signals in both axons and surrounding glial cells. This change in perception was initiated by the discovery of a spontaneously mutated mouse strain (called *Wld^S* or '*ola*'), in which peripheral nerves survive without any obvious changes for many weeks after transection. The full description of the local signals that initiate and control Wallerian degeneration is still wanting, yet it is clear that the enzyme system known as the ubiquitin–proteasome system (which includes ubiquitin regulatory enzyme UFD2 and the nicotinamide mononucleotide adenylyltransferase) plays a critical role. It was found that pharmacological inhibition of proteasomes delayed Wallerian degeneration in both peripheral nerves and optic nerve. Another important player involved in local signalling is represented by the Ca^{2+}-dependent proteases, calpains; inhibition of calpains or removal of Ca^{2+} delayed the onset and reduced the rate of Wallerian degeneration. This discovery opens important perspectives for treatment of naturally occurring neuropathies associated with degeneration of peripheral nerves, which are, for example, common in diabetes, some forms of HIV infection and chemotherapy.

9.3 Activation of microglia

Microglia are the immunocompetent cells specifically equipped to monitor the CNS environment. They represent the endogenous brain defence and immune system, which is responsible for CNS protection against all types of pathogenic factors. Microglial cells are not neural cells by their origin (see Chapter 3.5), nonetheless after invading and setting down in the CNS, they acquired a very specific phenotype, which clearly distinguish them from their ancestors, the blood-derived macrophages. The most important parts of this microglial phenotype are the very specialized appearance of resting microglial cells, and the peculiar complement of receptor molecules expressed by microglia. Microglial cells are endowed with

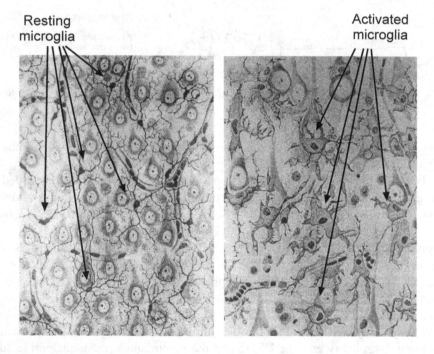

Figure 9.4 Resting and activated microglia as drawn by Pio del Rio-Hortega (1933). The left panel represents normal resting microglia, which were described by Rio-Hortega as 'the brain nerve cells have bodyguards which extend their tentacles in every direction, and hold back whatever might be noxious'. Right panel shows an encephalitic brain where these cells 'resemble voracious monsters and are valuable assistants in cleaning the tissue of whatever has damaged the nerve cells' (cited from Somjen GG (1988) Nervenkitt: notes on the history of the concept of neuroglia. *Glia* **1**, 2–9)

Resting 'ramified'
microglia

Activated microglia

Phagocytic or 'amoeboid'
microglia

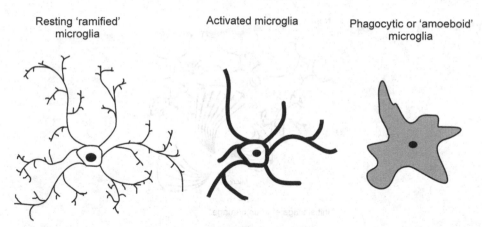

Figure 9.5 Schematic representation of microglial activation stages. The resting, or 'ramified' microglia has a small soma and several thin and long processes. Insult to the brain results in release of vascular, neuronal or astroglial factors (e.g. ATP, thrombin or cytokines), which trigger activation of microglia. The activated microglia is characterized by shorter and thicker processes and larger soma. The final stage of activation is represented by a phagocytic or 'amoeboid' microglia, which acts as a tissue microphage

both classical immunological receptors (e.g. complement receptors, cytokine and chemokine receptors, immunoglobulin receptors of the Fc family, thrombin and scavenger receptors) and classical neuro-ligand receptors (represented by glutamate, GABA, and P2X purinoreceptors).

Under physiological conditions microglia in the CNS exist in the 'resting' state (Figures 9.4, 9.5). The resting microglial cell is characterized by a small cell body and much elaborated thin processes, which send multiple branches and extend in all directions. Similar to astrocytes, every microglial cell has its own territory, about 30–15 μm wide; there is very little overlap between neighbouring cells. In essence the term 'resting' microglia can be somewhat misleading, as microglia in unperturbed brain are far from being quiescent. The processes of resting microglial cells are constantly moving through its territory; this is a relatively rapid movement with a speed ~1.2–1.5 μm/min. At the same time microglial processes also constantly send out and retract small protrusions, which can grow and shrink by 2–3 μm/min. The movement of microglial processes does not have any manifest pattern; the microglia seem to be randomly scanning through their domains (Figure 9.6). Considering the velocity of this movement, the brain parenchyma can be completely scanned by microglial processes every several hours. The motility of the processes is not affected by neuronal firing, but it is sensitive to activators (ATP and its analogues) and inhibitors of purinoreceptors. Focal neuronal damage induces a rapid (~1.5 μm) and concerted movement of many microglial processes towards the site of lesion, and very soon the latter is completely surrounded by these processes. This injury-induced motility is also governed, at least in part, by activation of purinoreceptors; it is also sensitive to the inhibition of gap junctions,

Normal conditions

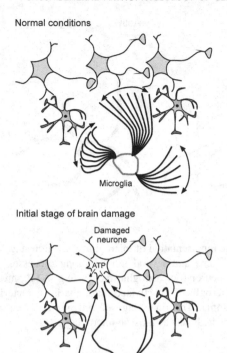

Microglia

Initial stage of brain damage

Damaged
neurone

ATP

Microglia

Figure 9.6 Microglial cells constantly scan their territories and send their processes towards the site of injury. In the resting condition every microglial cell occupies a distinct territory. Processes of resting microglial cells are constantly moving, scanning this territory for possible damage signals. In the case of local insult microglial processes rapidly move to the source of the damage signal; the latter is most likely represented by ATP that stimulates microglial process movement through activation of metabotropic P2Y purinoreceptors

which are present in astrocytes, but not in microglia; inhibition of gap junctions also affects physiological motility of astroglial processes. Therefore, it appears that astrocytes signal to the microglia by releasing ATP (and possibly some other molecules) through connexin hemichannels. All in all, microglial processes act as a very sophisticated and fast scanning system. This system can, by virtue of receptors residing in the microglial cell plasmalemma, immediately detect injury and initiate the process of active response, which eventually triggers the full blown microglial activation.

When a brain insult is detected by microglial cells, they launch a specific programme that results in the gradual transformation of resting microglia into a phagocyte; this process is generally referred to as 'microglial activation' and proceeds through several steps (Figures 9.4 and 9.5). The first stage of microglial activation produces 'normally' activated or reactive microglia. During this transition, resting microglia retract their processes, which become fewer and much thicker, increase the size of their cell bodies, change the expression of various enzymes and receptors, and begin to produce immune response molecules. At this activated stage, some microglial cells return into a proliferative mode, and microglial numbers around the lesion site start to multiply. Finally, microglial cells become motile, and using amoeboid-like movements they gather around sites of insult. If the damage persists and CNS cells begin to die, microglial cells undergo further transformation and become phagocytes. This is, naturally, a rather sketchy account of complex and highly coordinated changes which occur in microglial cells; the process of activation is gradual and most likely many sub-states exist on the way from resting to phagocytic microglia. Furthermore, activated microglial cells may display quite heterogeneous properties in different types of pathology and in different parts of the brain.

The precise nature of the initial signal that triggers the process of microglial activation is not fully understood; it may be associated either with withdrawal of some molecules (the 'off-signal') released during normal CNS activity, or by the appearance of abnormal molecules or abnormal concentrations of otherwise physiologically present molecules (the 'on-signal'). Both types of signalling can provide microglia with relevant information about the status of brain parenchyma within their territorial domain.

The 'off-signals' that may indicate deterioration in neural networks are not yet fully characterized. A good example of this type of communication is represented by neuronal firing: depression of the latter affects neighbouring microglia, turning them if not into an activated, then into an 'alerted' state – in response to blockade of neuronal activity microglial cells start to up-regulate several immunocompetent molecules. In fact these 'off-signals' can be defensively important as they allow microglia to sense some disturbances even if the nature of the damaging factor cannot be identified.

The 'on-signalling' is conveyed by a wide array of molecules, either associated with cell damage or with foreign matter invading the brain. In particular, damaged neurones can release high amounts of ATP, nucleotides, neuropeptides, growth factors, neurotransmitters, etc. Practically all of these factors can be sensed by microglia (which are endowed with a remarkable array of receptors, see Table 5.1 and Chapter 5) and trigger activation. It might well be that different molecules can activate various subprogrammes of this routine, regulating therefore the speed and degree and peculiar features of microglial activation. Some of these molecules can carry both 'off' and 'on' signals: for example low concentrations of ATP may be indicative of normal on-going synaptic activity, whereas high concentrations signal cell damage. Microglia are also capable of sensing disturbances in brain metabolism: for example, accumulation of ammonia, which follows grave metabolic failures (e.g. during hepatic encephalopathy) can activate microglial cells either directly or via intermediates such as NO or ATP.

Astroglial cells are also capable of releasing a variety of molecules that can activate microglia; this is especially characteristic of activated astroglia, which can up-regulate the synthesis and begin to release biologically active molecules. Microglial cells can also be activated by signals released from their sister cells, which have already undergone activation. An important activator signal is conveyed by molecules arriving with infectious agents, e.g. by lypopolysaccharides, forming the bacterial cellular wall, by prions, or by viral components, such as g120 protein from HIV. Finally, microglia can be activated by a number of molecules which can infiltrate the brain following damage to the blood–brain barrier, e.g. by coagulation factors, immunoglobulins, albumin, thrombin etc.

Intracellularly, most of the 'on' signals produce elevations in $[Ca^{2+}]_i$, the amplitude and shape of which vary significantly depending on the type and concentration of molecule/receptor complex involved. Most likely, these variabilities of the Ca^{2+} signals are instrumental for information encoding, although the precise nature of this type of informational processing remains unknown.

Activation that follows the recognition of damage signals can be a very rapid process indeed. The initial changes in cellular biochemistry occur within minutes after the presenting signal, and the full activation of microglial cells can follow within several hours. Activated microglial cells change their physiological and biochemical properties considerably. First, activated microglia start to up-regulate potassium channels, initially K_{ir} and then delayed K^+ channels. Second, activated microglia can change the repertoire and levels of expression of numerous receptors, e.g. by down-regulating 'neuronal' receptors and up-regulating the 'immunocompetent' ones. Furthermore, activated microglial cells alter their biochemistry, by stimulating the synthesis of numerous enzymes. Finally, microglial cells change their motility as they gather at the site of damage, first by sending their processes and then by appearing there in soma.

All these changes allow the execution of the primary function of microglia – defence. This function requires the ability to rapidly attack and kill the invader; subsequently, the remnants of the aggressor, its victims and the collateral damage must be effectively removed. Thus, activated microglial cells are fully equipped with cytotoxic tools, like reactive oxygen species, or NO (most notably the NO system is absent in human microglia, although it is fully operative in rodents), or indeed the cytokines and chemokines. Not only, however, do activated microglial cells aim to destroy the foreign cells, but also to assist neurones in overcoming the damage. In line with this, microglial cells express and release various growth factors (NGF, BDNF, NT-3, NT-4 etc.). Microglial activation often leads to high expression of glutamate transporter (GLT-1), which assists in clearing the excess of glutamate. It has been suggested that microglial cells after arriving at the location of damage, can selectively remove excitatory glutamatergic synapses (so-called 'synaptic stripping'), which further limits glutamate release into compromised brain regions. Finally, microglial cells produce an incredible array of immunocompetent molecules, which include numerous interleukins (IL-1α/β; IL-3, IL-6, IL-8, IL-10, IL-12, IL-15, IL-18), tumour necrosis factor α, interferon inducing factor (IGIF), inflammatory proteins, transforming growth factor TGFβ, etc. All these molecules regulate the inflammatory processes and control the immune response of the brain.

Many of these, such as TGFβ, are also important regulators of astrogliosis and are important in the orchestration of glial scar formation.

Microglial activation is a reversible process (except the final, phagocytic, stage), which occurs when the pathological factor is defeated. The nature of the signals regulating the deactivation of microglia is unknown. Most likely, the waning of pathological stimulation may be sufficient, although some active 'terminating' message is not excluded. Some *in vitro* experiments have shown the existence of certain astrocyte-derived factors that may initiate deactivation of microglia.

The final transmutation from activated microglia into a phagocytic one is also initiated by factors released from dying or already dead neurones or astrocytes. The nature of these 'death signals' is not very clear; it seems likely that vanishing cells can release certain chemoattractants (e.g. phosphatidylserine and lysophosphatidylcholine), which can initiate the ultimate transformation of microglial cells into phagocytes; the latter engulf and devour the remnants of dying cells. Importantly, the actual killing of neurones by microglia is confined to the damaged area, and, normally, it does not extend to undamaged areas. When this constraint fails, however, activated microglia may assume the role of brain destroyer, which does happen in certain pathological conditions.

9.3.1 Pathological potential of activated microglia

As is the case for macrophages in many body systems, microglia are capable of providing both protection and destruction. The exaggerated or prolonged activation of microglial cells can be detrimental to the brain. In certain cases, the pathological activation of microglia may have a decisive input into the pathological developments. This may happen, for example, in infectious diseases, in particular in certain types of bacterial infection or in prion diseases (see Chapter 10). Similarly, chronic neurodegenerative diseases (e.g. Alzheimer's or Parkinson's disease – Chapter 10) may underlie the long-lasting over-activation of microglial cells, which subsequently may produce neuronal or astroglial death.

10
Glia and Diseases of the Nervous System

10.1 Alexander's disease

Alexander's disease (AxD), described by Stewart Alexander in 1949, is a fatal, albeit rare, disease that strikes infants and young adults; AxD is the only example of a primary disease of astrocytes, which is associated with their intrinsic malfunction. The histological hallmark of AxD is the presence of *Rosenthal fibres* in astrocytes, which are cytoplasmic inclusions, formed by GFAP in association with stress proteins (such as α- and β-crystallin and heat shock protein 27). Infantile and juvenile AxD is mostly caused by mis-sense mutations of the GFAP gene; these aberrant genes are absent in parents, and therefore represent de-novo dominant GFAP gene mutations. Very rarely, AxD can be diagnosed in adults, but the aetiology remains unclear. Infantile AxD usually becomes manifest around six months of age and the symptoms include head enlargement, convulsions, pyramidal symptoms, and muscle weakness. The infants die within two to four years after the onset of the disease. The juvenile form (onset ~nine years, average survival eight years after diagnosis) is characterized by progressive paresis. The precise nature of AxD pathology is not defined, but the progression of the disease is determined by rapidly developing demyelination. There are suggestions that AxD development may result from permanent disruption of the blood brain barrier (as Rosenthal fibres tend to accumulate in endfeet, both in perivascular and pial zones), and overall malfunction of astrocytes.

10.2 Spreading depression

The spreading depression of electric activity in the cerebral cortex, initially described by Aristide Leào in 1944, is a wave of cellular depolarization, which travels through the grey matter at a velocity of about 1.5 to 7.5 mm/min. This propagating wave of depolarization can be triggered by local massive increases

Glial Neurobiology: A Textbook Alexei Verkhratsky and Arthur Butt
© 2007 John Wiley & Sons, Ltd ISBN 978-0-470-01564-3 (HB); 978-0-470-51740-6 (PB)

in extracellular K^+ concentration and/or glutamate, which are the consequences of exaggerated focal electrical activity or mechanical or ischaemic injury. The most striking features of spreading depression are the rapid propagating elevation of extracellular K^+ concentration up to $80\,mM$; a dramatic ($\sim$10 times) decrease in extracellular Ca^{2+} concentration and propagating shrinkage of the extracellular space by up to 50 per cent. These changes have complex kinetics, and begin with an initial slight elevation in extracellular K^+, which is followed by a regenerative steep increase in $[K^+]_o$, decrease in $[Ca^{2+}]_o$ and shrinkage of the extracellular space. During this period of excessive rise in $[K^+]_o$, Na^+, Ca^{2+} and Cl^- ions enter the cells, which rapidly eliminates neuronal excitability. In the meantime, astroglial cells become alkaline, most likely due to the activity of bicarbonate transporter. Elevation of extracellular K^+ concentration lasts for one to two minutes, after which the cells repolarize, and all ion gradients are normalized (the recovery period). Neurones regain their excitability within the subsequent three to five minutes, and the whole wave of spreading depression can be repeated after another 10 minutes (which reflects the refractory period). Spreading depression waves in normal tissue do not result in any cell damage, although repetitive incidences of spreading depression may activate microglia and induce reactive astrogliosis in its mild form; both processes seem to be fully reversible. In conditions of brain ischaemia, however, spreading depression may increase the area of cellular damage (see Chapter 10.3).

There is much evidence linking the development of spreading depression with astroglial networks; particularly important are the demonstration of the effective inhibition of spreading depression by pharmacological inhibition of gap junctions and the discovery of circulating currents passing through the glial syncytium during a course of spreading depolarization. An apparent similarity between propagating astroglial calcium waves and the propagation of spreading depression led to a hypothesis of a triggering role for the former; this remains controversial, however; as in mouse neocortex, for example, it was possible to pharmacologically dissociate astroglial calcium waves and spreading depression. Nonetheless, the leading role played by astrocytes in the development of spreading depression remains firm; although the underlying mechanisms require further elaboration. The pathological potential of spreading depression also requires further attention; at present it is implicated in the developments of migraine and brain ischaemic damage.

10.3   Stroke and ischaemia

It is a truth generally acknowledged that disruption of the blood flow in the brain causes considerable damage and death of neuronal cells. Generally speaking, the disruption of blood flow can be caused either by blood vessel rupture, which results in *haemorrhage*, or by a restriction of blood supply to the brain or parts of the brain, commonly referred to as *brain ischaemia*, due to vascular occlusion (because of thrombosis or embolism), or to a systemic decrease in blood supply (for example, associated with heart failure). As a consequence, brain ischaemia can be either global, or focal, the latter corresponding to a *stroke*. Focal ischaemia triggers local cell death, the localization and volume of the damage being determined by anatomical localization of vessel occlusion. Often, the conditions of focal ischaemia are transient as the blood flow can be restored when the vessel blockage is removed; the restored blood flow results in *reperfusion* of the damaged area; this can be potentially damaging because of the production of reactive oxygen species. The pathogenesis of ischaemia is associated with the limitation of oxygen supply (hypoxia or anoxia), as well as with restrictions in supply of metabolic substrates.

Global ischaemia develops as a consequence of transient heart arrest. This leads to an almost immediate cessation of the cerebral blood flow from a normal ∼8 ml/g/min to zero. About 10–15 seconds of global brain ischaemia results in loss of consciousness, while electrical activity of the brain disappears 30–40 seconds after the beginning of circulatory arrest. Global ischaemia lasting for more than 10 min at normal temperature is lethal for humans. On a cellular level short periods of global ischaemia trigger delayed selective neuronal death, while, at least initially, astrocytes survive and become activated.

The development of focal ischaemic damage to brain tissue has a much more complicated kinetics. The cessation of, or a considerable decrease in, local cerebral blood flow triggers the onset of infarction. The *core* (Figure 10.1) of the infarction zone (were the blood flow rates are reduced below 1ml/g/min) is the region of pan-necrosis of all cells including neurones, astrocytes, oligodendrocytes and ependymal cells. The infarction core is surrounded by a zone of reduced circulation (with rates 2–4 ml/g/min) known as the '*ischaemic penumbra*' (Figure 10.1). The penumbra contains viable cells, albeit with compromised metabolism and function. The infarction core is formed very rapidly, within minutes and hours after initiation of the stroke, a much slower process of expansion of the infarction zone follows; this process developing over many hours and even days.

Glial cells are intimately involved in the CNS response to the ischaemia. Astrocytes, in particular, to a very large extent determine the progression and outcome of focal ischaemia. Importantly, astroglial cells have a dual role in the reactions to ischaemia, as they may either reduce or exacerbate neuronal damage, depending on the depth of ischaemia and timing relative to the moment of insult.

10.3.1 Glial cell death during ischaemia

The cells located within the infarction core region rapidly undergo an anoxic depolarization; as a result neurones cease to be electrically excitable and lose their ability to maintain transmembrane ion gradients. This results in a considerable Na^+ and Ca^{2+} influx into the cells accompanied by a substantial K^+ efflux, so that very

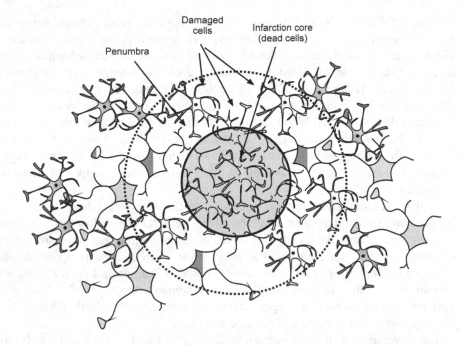

Figure 10.1 Histology of focal ischaemic damage of the brain. The focal ischaemic damage (or stroke) comprises the central zone of the infarction core, where all the cells are dead and a much larger surrounding zone of penumbra, which contains partially damaged cells. The progression of the penumbra and increase of the infarction core may take several days and can be determined by propagation of death signals through astroglial syncytium

soon (within minutes) the extracellular ion concentration deteriorates severely: e.g. in the grey matter $[K^+]_o$ rises to 40–80 mM, whereas $[Na^+]_o$ and $[Ca^{2+}]_o$ decline to 60 mM and 0.2–0.5 mM respectively (Figure 10.2). Massive Ca^{2+} influx triggers release of glutamate from neuronal terminals, which further amplifies the vicious circle by '*glutamate excitotoxicity*' (Figure 10.3). Simultaneously, the extracellular milieu becomes acidic (the extracellular pH drops to 6.5). These events almost immediately kill the neurones and most likely the glial cells too. In the penumbra, the extent of cellular changes is much less pronounced – neurones lose electrical excitability, yet all the cells retain their ion homeostasis and continue to survive, although their cytosol is often acidified, they swell, and protein synthesis and general metabolism are inhibited.

Neurones and oligodendrocytes are the most vulnerable and sensitive to ischaemic shock; astrocytes are generally more resilient. The initial cell death, which follows the stroke, is associated with 'glutamate excitotoxicity'; massive release of glutamate in the core region leads to the sustained activation of neuronal NMDA receptors, which results in Ca^{2+} influx; simultaneously neuronal depolarization opens voltage-gated Ca^{2+} channels, which add to the Ca^{2+} entry. At the end, neurones become overloaded with Ca^{2+}, which strains metabolic processes.

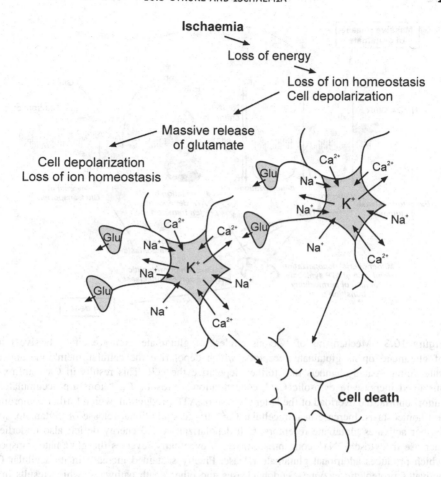

Figure 10.2 Mechanisms of ischaemic cell death: Ischaemic cell death is initiated by compromised energy production, which in turn triggers loss of ion homeostasis and depolarization of the injured neural cell. This depolarization leads to a massive release of glutamate, which further depolarizes the injured cells and the cells in their immediate vicinity; this induces additional glutamate release thus establishing the vicious circle of glutamate excitotoxicity. Opening of NMDA glutamate receptors and depolarization induces uncontrolled Ca^{2+} entry in the cytosol, which (a) compromises mitochondria and ATP production and (b) activates numerous proteolytic enzymes and caspase-dependent cell death pathways. This results in necrotic cell death, cell disintegration and release of cellular content into the brain parenchyma, which acts as a damage signal for neighbouring neurones and glia

A substantial part of the Ca^{2+} is accumulated by mitochondria, which eventually depolarize. This in turn blocks ATP synthesis and opens a highly permeable mitochondrial channel known as the *permeability transition pore*; this process signals the demise of mitochondria and the complete disintegration of cellular homeostasis. Persistently elevated $[Ca^{2+}]_i$ activates numerous proteolytic enzymes and initiates necrotic neuronal death (Figure 10.3).

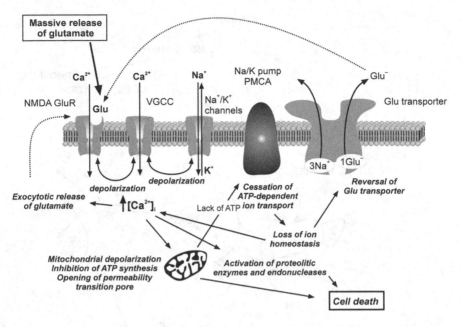

Figure 10.3 Mechanisms of 'vicious circles' of glutamate excitotoxicity. Massive release of glutamate opens glutamate receptors, which depolarize the cellular membrane and activate voltage-gated channels that further depolarize the cell. This results in Ca^{2+} influx and sustained increase in cytosolic Ca^{2+} concentration. Cytosolic Ca^{2+} ions are accumulated by mitochondria; the overload of the latter Ca^{2+} stops ATP production, which further compromises ion homeostasis. Increase in intracellular Ca^{2+} triggers additional release of glutamate, which further activates glutamate receptors. Cell depolarization and energy deficit also underlie the increase in cytosolic Na^+ concentration, which eventually reverses the glutamate transporter, which produces additional glutamate release. Finally sustained increase in intracellular Ca^{2+} activates proteolytic enzymes, endonucleases and other death pathways, which results in cell demise

Oligodendrocyte precursors and mature oligodendrocytes are also very sensitive to ischaemia and glutamate excitotoxicity. Even short periods of anoxia/ischaemia cause complete loss of oligodendroglial ion homeostasis, and a very substantial $[Ca^{2+}]_i$ elevation. The overload of oligodendrocytes with Ca^{2+} triggers oxidative stress and mitochondrial damage, with subsequent induction of necrosis or apoptosis, depending on the intensity of the insult.

Initiation of a toxic Ca^{2+} load in oligodendrocytes results from activation of several neurotransmitter receptors, and particularly glutamate receptors of AMPA/kainate and (at least in some brain regions) NMDA type. Glutamate concentration around ischaemic axons can rise very rapidly; axoplasm contains ~1 mM of glutamate, and the axolemma is endowed with Na^+/glutamate transporters. Loss of ion homeostasis triggered by ischaemia causes acute axonal depolarization (due to $[K^+]_o$ increase) and substantial elevation in axoplasmic

Na^+; these changes result in reversal of the Na^+/glutamate transporter and massive release of glutamate. Glutamate in turn triggers Ca^{2+} entry into oligo-dendroglial cells: the latter do not express the GluR2 AMPA receptor subunit (see Chapter 5.3.1), and this renders their AMPA receptors Ca^{2+} permeable; similarly Ca^{2+} also can pass through kainate receptors; recent data also indicate that at least some oligodendrocytes express NMDA receptors, which can be activated during ischaemia. Oligodendrocyte precursors, which have particularly high levels of AMPA/kainate receptor expression, appear the most vulnerable to glutamate toxicity. Interestingly, exposure to glutamate can directly destroy the myelin sheath; this involves Ca^{2+} influx through NMDA receptors, which are localized to myelin sheaths, whereas ionotropic AMPA receptors appear to be localized to the cell bodies and may mediate cell death. Indeed Ca^{2+} influx into the compact myelin affected by ischaemia has been directly demonstrated in imaging experiments; moreover antagonists to NMDA receptors prevented ischaemia-induced deterioration of myelin. Another important pathway for $[Ca^{2+}]_i$ elevation is associated with Ca^{2+} release from the ER store activated by depolarization of oligodendrocyte membrane, which results from acute elevation in extracellular $[K^+]$, triggered by ischaemia (depolarization-induced Ca^{2+} release through RyRs – see Chapter 5.4).

Astrocytes generally are less sensitive to glutamate excitotoxicity. Astroglial cultures readily survive relatively prolonged periods (up to several hours) of oxygen and/or glucose deprivation. *In vivo,* however, astrocyte sensitivity to ischaemic insults seems to be much higher. Many, but not all astroglial cells in hippocampus survive brief (~10 min) periods of ischaemia (which is enough to kill a very significant number of neurones), yet longer cessation of blood flow causes prominent astrocytic death. White matter astrocytes seem to be even more vulnerable: astroglial cells in the optic nerve begin to die within 10 to 20 minutes after the onset of ischaemia.

Nonetheless, astroglial cells can survive for long periods of time in the penumbra. In the latter, the reduced blood flow still delivers relatively high amounts of glucose, which can be utilized by astrocytes through anaerobic glycolysis. This, however, produces lactate, which in turn promotes acidosis. Importantly, astroglia are rather sensitive to acidification of their environment: lowering of pH to ~6.6 completely inhibits astroglial ATP production and very rapidly (in about 15 minutes *in vitro*) kills astrocytes. Interestingly, hyperglycaemia exacerbates growth of the infarction core, most likely through intensifying anaerobic glycolysis and increasing acidosis. At the same time astrocytes are also vulnerable to reactive oxygen species (ROS), which can be produced in large quantities during reperfusion; ROS induce cell death through mitochondrial depolarization and opening of the permeability transition pore. One of the early consequences of astroglial injury is the disruption of their distal processes; the phenomenon described a century ago by Alzheimer and Ramón y Cajal as *clasmatodendrosis* ('fragmentation of dendrites' from the Greek 'clasmato' 'κλασματο' – fragment, piece broken off).

10.3.2 Astroglia protect the brain against ischaemia

Notwithstanding the detrimental effects of profound ischaemia on astroglial cells, the latter still remain the most resistant elements of neural circuits, which protect the brain against injury (Figure 10.4).

First and foremost, astrocytes form the main barrier against glutamate excitotoxicity. Astroglial cells, by virtue of numerous transporters (see Chapters 5.7 and 7.8) expressed in their membrane, act as the main sink for the glutamate in the CNS. Furthermore, the astroglial ability to maintain anaerobic ATP production is of great help, as it allows sustained glutamate transport in hypoxic conditions. Astroglial protection against glutamate excitotoxicity became very obvious from *in vitro* experiments: withdrawal of astrocytes from neuronal cultures led to a 100-times increase in the vulnerability of neurones to glutamate infusion. Similarly, genetic down-regulation of glial glutamate transporters exacerbates brain ischaemic damage.

Second, astrocytes are powerful scavengers of ROS; the latter being one of the main mediators of ischaemic brain injury. Astrocytes contain high concentrations of glutathione and ascorbate, which are the principal antioxidants in the brain. Ascorbate is a component of neuronal–astroglial exchange, as neurones release oxidized ascorbate, which is accumulated by astrocytes, and subsequently converted into ascorbate ready for a new cycle of ROS scavenging. The ability of astrocytes to protect neurones against ROS has been clearly demonstrated

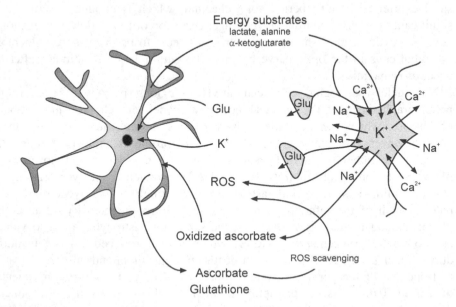

Figure 10.4 Mechanisms of astroglia-dependent neuroprotection. Astroglial cells act as the main sink for glutamate, buffer extracellular potassium, provide neurones with energy substrates and serve as the main source of reactive oxygen species scavengers

in vitro: neuronal–astroglial cultures were much more resistant to injury produced by superoxide or hydrogen peroxide, as compared to purified neuronal cultures.

Third, anaerobic metabolism sustained by astrocytes in hypoxic conditions produces several intermediate substrates, such as lactate, alanine and α-ketoglutarate, which can be fed to neurones and support energy production in conditions of glucose deprivation.

Fourth, astrocytic networks are involved in potassium buffering through either K^+ uptake or K^+ spatial buffering (Chapter 7.7.1), which by removing the excess of potassium may slow down neuronal depolarization and depolarization-induced glutamate release.

Finally, in the more delayed stages of the infarction, the process of reactive astrogliosis leads to an appearance of a protective astrocyte wall, which isolates the damaged area. Subsequently, the reactive astrocytes produce a scar that fills the core necrotic area.

10.3.3 Astrocytes may exacerbate brain damage upon ischaemia

Astrocytes, however, may act not only as protectors of the brain; in certain conditions (especially upon severe insults) astroglial cells may exacerbate the cell damage, contributing to several vicious circles triggered by the stroke. First of all, the astroglial involvement in controlling brain glutamate concentration is double edged. The ability of astrocytes to remove glutamate from the extracellular space leads to glutamate accumulation in their cytosol in very high concentrations (up to 10 mM). Upon severe hypoxic/hypoglycaemic conditions astroglial cells may turn from being the sink for glutamate to being the main source of the latter. Astrocytes can release glutamate by several mechanisms (see Chapter 5.6) which are triggered in ischaemia: (1) reversal of glutamate transporters can be caused by ATP depletion accompanied with an increase in intracellular Na^+ concentration and cell depolarization; (2) elevation of $[Ca^{2+}]_i$ in astrocytes, which follows the ischaemic insult, may trigger the release of glutamate stored in vesicles; (3) acidosis and lowering of extracellular Ca^{2+} concentration can open glutamate-permeable hemichannels; (4) ATP released in high concentrations by dying and disintegrating neurones can open astroglial $P2X_7$ purinoreceptors, which also allow glutamate release; and (5) brain oedema can activate volume-sensitive channels, which also allow passage of glutamate.

The second important pathological role of astrocytes is associated with a progression of the infarction core through the penumbra. This expansion of the death zone is a slow process, which may proceed for several days after the initial insult. It is more than likely that growth of the infarct zone into the penumbra, or alternatively containing the infarct zone within its initial borders, is a highly complex process, which involves different cellular mechanisms. The importance of the core–penumbra interactions is also obvious because this process determines the final extent of brain damage.

The slow progression of damage spread through the ischaemic penumbra implicates specific signalling processes propagating from the infarction core towards the surrounding tissue. Signalling through neuronal network can be excluded, as neuronal excitability is lost after even a mild reduction of cerebral blood flow. The alternative route for propagation of death signals may involve the astroglial syncytium. This scenario begins with the generation of aberrant $[Ca^{2+}]_i$ waves in an astrocyte which may in turn evoke the distant release of glutamate from astrocytes beyond the ischaemic focus. Thus, a propagating wave of glutamate release from astrocytes can contribute to the extension of infarction (Figure 10.5).

The second route for infarction expansion is associated with spreading depression, which often occurs in the penumbra (Chapter 10.2). The spreading depression waves originate at the very border between the necrotic core and the ischaemic penumbra, and these waves are initiated by high extracellular K^+ concentration present around the core. The spreading depression wave occurs as often as every 10–15 minutes, which is determined by the refractory period of the cells in the penumbra. There is a fundamental difference between spreading depression in normal brain tissue and in the compromised ischaemic penumbra. The cells in penumbra retain their ion homeostasis, and therefore each wave of spreading

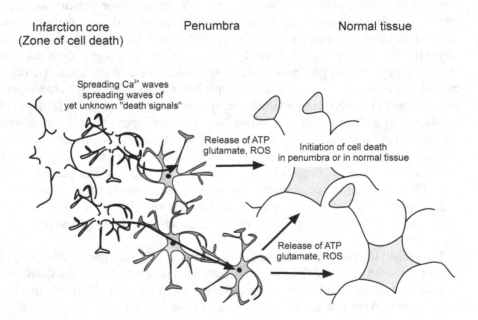

Infarction core   Penumbra   Normal tissue
(Zone of cell death)

Spreading Ca²⁺ waves
spreading waves of
yet unknown "death signals"

Release of ATP
glutamate, ROS   Initiation of cell death
in penumbra or in normal tissue

Release of ATP
glutamate, ROS

Figure 10.5 Astrocytes may exacerbate infarction progression through the penumbra by propagating Ca^{2+} waves or by propagating 'death signals'. Death signals may travel through the astroglial syncytium, triggering injury to cells distant to the site of the infarction. See the text for detailed explanation

depression results in further imbalance between the energy requirement of the depolarized tissue and the energy supply; this imbalance leads to cell death. As a result, there is a direct correlation between the number of spreading depression waves and the spread of necrotic area into the penumbra. Metabolic imbalance also determines the longer duration and longer recovery of spreading depression in ischaemic penumbra. The spreading depression waves propagate from the ischaemic region to the healthy tissue, causing some functional disturbances, although this does not result in any cell death outside the borders of ischaemic tissue.

The extension of the necrotic zone through the penumbra may demarcate the primary extension of astroglial failure, which in turn depends on a variety of factors. For example, the extent of the circulation breakdown would determine the relative activity of glycolysis, and hence production of lactate and accumulation of protons in the extracellular space. Profound extracellular acidification will in turn induce astrocytic collapse. This process can be further exacerbated by accumulation of extracellular K^+ ions and subsequent depolarization, accompanying for example the wave of spreading depression. At the same time release of glutamate by astrocytes in the penumbra can kill neighbouring neurones and produce even further accumulation of K^+ and secondary release of glutamate and ATP. At the same time increases in $[K^+]_o$ would initiate astroglial swelling, which will reduce the extracellular space, hence further increasing concentrations of K^+ and glutamate in the latter, and further obstructing circulation. In other words, the very same mechanisms that protect neurones during ischaemic stress, may also participate in extending the damage; this happens when the astroglial capacity for survival in ischaemic conditions is exhausted, which in turn activates several vicious positive feedback loops, that result in cell death and in extension of the necrotic zone through ischaemic penumbra. All in all, the stroke should never be considered as a primary neuronal disease, as indeed the outcome of focal brain ischaemia is directly determined by astroglial performance.

10.3.4 Oligodendrocytes and microglia in stroke

Death of oligodendrocytes leads to axonal disintegration; as mentioned above oligodendroglia are particularly vulnerable to focal ischaemia. Strokes located in the white matter may therefore trigger particularly dangerous disruptions of nerve fibres and lead to severe functional disabilities (such as focal insults in the internal capsule). Microglial cells are also activated during brain ischaemia; their activation is associated with the release of numerous immunocompetent molecules, which can have either beneficial or detrimental effects. Profound activation of microglial cells may turn them into phagocytes; the latter can launch a direct attack on neural cells thus contributing to the expansion of the necrotic zone.

10.4   Cytotoxic brain oedema

Homeostatic regulation of brain volume and water content is of paramount importance for its function. Brain size is limited by the skull, and therefore even minute
increases in brain volume lead to an increase in intracranial pressure and compression damage of neural tissue. Water redistribution between brain compartments
compromises the extracellular space with similarly grave consequences. Brain
oedema is in essence a collapse of brain volume/water regulation, which exists
in two forms – *vascular* and *cellular* (also known as *cytotoxic*); vascular oedema
is a consequence of disruption of the blood–brain barrier, which triggers water
flow into the tissue, whereas cellular oedema is a redistribution of water into
cellular compartments, which does not necessarily affect total volume of the brain
parenchyma.

Physiologically, astrocytes are capable of rapidly responding to changes in extracellular osmotic pressure by an initial swelling and consequent regulatory volume
decrease; this response is regulated by ion and water movements (Chapter 7.9).
In pathology, these mechanisms are compromised, which hampers the ability of
astrocytes to maintain their volume and water content.

Cellular oedema is primarily astroglial pathology, as astrocytes are capable
of large volume changes due to water fluxes. Indeed many brain insults, such
as ischaemia or acute trauma, result in rapid swelling of astrocytes, which is

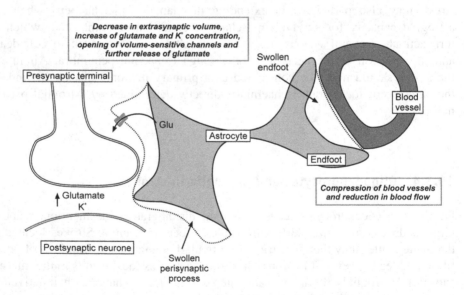

Figure 10.6 Pathological potential of astroglial swelling. Astroglial swelling decreases extracellular volume, hence increasing concentration of neurotransmitters and damage signals in the
interstitium and compresses brain capillaries, further compromising circulation in the damaged
area

accompanied by a significant increase in astroglial surface area. Astroglial swelling can trigger numerous secondary effects, which exacerbate the brain damage (Figure 10.6). In particular, swelling of perivascular astrocytes and astrocyte endfeet may compress brain vessels and limit circulation. This compression, for example, accounts for noncomplete filling of brain vessels during reperfusion following focal ischaemia; this is known as the *no-reflow* phenomenon. Swelling of astrocytes can result in opening of volume-regulated ion channels, permeable to glutamate and other excitatory amino acids; release of the latter can induce or exacerbate excitotoxic cell death. Prominent swelling of astrocytes can severely reduce the extracellular space volume with obvious consequences of increased concentration of extracellular glutamate and K^+ ions. In fact, a several fold reduction in extracellular space can increase the concentration of the latter to excitotoxic levels.

10.4.1 Ischaemic oedema

Astroglial swelling becomes apparent within 30 minutes of the onset of focal ischaemia. This swelling is quite prominent and water redistribution into the astroglial cells may reduce the total extracellular volume by 50–75 per cent. The initiation of astrocyte swelling upon ischaemia most likely is associated with increased levels of glutamate and K^+, which being pumped into astrocytes, trigger the osmotic overload of the latter. This activates water influx through aquaporins, abundantly expressed in astrocyte membranes, and results in the dramatic increase in their volume.

10.4.2 Traumatic oedema

Posttraumatic astroglial swelling occurs within 30–40 minutes after trauma, and mechanistically is very similar to ischaemic swelling, with extracellular increases in glutamate and K^+ concentration taking the lead pathological roles. Posttraumatic oedema is complicated, however, by the presence of a strong vascular component, which underlies water influx into the brain through a compromised blood–brain barrier.

10.4.3 Hepatic encephalopathy

Brain oedema frequently accompanies liver failure and represents cytotoxic, cellular oedema in its pure form. As a consequence of intoxication, astrocytes are primarily affected, and they are the only cells which show prominent morphological changes in postmortem analysis. Astroglial swelling is proportional to the blood levels of ammonia (which increases following liver breakdown) and results from intracellular accumulation of organic osmolytes, with subsequent collapse of volume-regulating mechanisms.

10.4.4   Hyponatremia

Decreases in plasma sodium levels below 120 mM, which occurs following disruption of kidney electrolyte handling, results in the rapid development of brain oedema, which is the main cause of mortality. Disruption of electrolyte secretion/reuptake in kidneys can be triggered by a variety of clinical factors, including endocrine pathology (e.g. hypothyroidism or overproduction of antidiuretic hormone), heart failure, HIV infection etc.

Hypernatremia induces hypo-osmotic shock in the brain tissue, which in turn triggers prominent swelling of astrocytes and neuronal dendrites. In mild cases, transport of electrolytes and osmolytes may fully compensate for disruption of osmotic gradients.

10.5   Neurodegenerative diseases

10.5.1   Normal ageing

Ageing of the brain is manifested by cognitive decline. For many years, this decline in the most important of brain functions was associated with neuronal loss, as it was believed that senescence is inevitably associated with neuronal death. Recent investigations, however, have shown that physiological brain ageing (i.e. in the absence of evident neurodegenerative pathology) is not associated with appreciable neuronal loss. On the other hand, glial cells are affected in physiological brain ageing. In astrocytes, advanced age initiates conditions similar to a mild reactive gliosis. Astroglial cells from old brain have higher expression of GFAP and the glial calcium binding protein S100. There are some indications that the number of astrocytes in aged brain can be increased by as much as 20 per cent, although these estimates require more precise definition. Overall, numbers of oligodendrocytes and microglia are not changed in aged brain, although the number of activated microglial cells is significantly increased.

10.5.2   Post-stroke dementia

Post-stroke dementia (PSD) is currently defined as any dementia occurring after stroke. The overall statistic is striking as the incidence of stroke doubles the risk of dementia. There is also a direct link between stroke and development of Alzheimer's disease; although the latter is responsible only for part of the eventually developed dementias; the fraction of patients with Alzheimer's disease accounts for 20–60 per cent of those with PSD.

Brain defects that develop after stroke are directly associated with glial cells, as both astrocytes and microglia determine the size of the infarction, and through permissive astrogliosis they determine posttraumatic remodelling and regeneration of brain regions, which were not put to death by infarction (Chapter 9.1). Therefore, new therapeutic strategies aimed at glial cells may significantly affect the functional outcome and prevalence of PSD.

A particular type of post-stroke dementia is represented by *Binswanger's disease*, (or subcortical dementia), which is a form of vascular dementia characterized by diffuse white matter lesions; it leads to progressive loss of memory, cognition and behavioural adaptation. The infarct occurring in white matter triggers progressive death of oligodendrocytes, activation of microglia and degeneration of axons. The primary pathological steps most likely are associated with ischaemic death of oligodendrocytes.

Another relatively frequent and grim outcome of brain ischaemia-related disease is represented by *periventricular leucomalacia*; a condition that causes diffuse cerebral white matter injury. This occurs mostly in prematurely (<32 weeks) born infants; an especially high incidence (up to 20 per cent) of periventricular leucomalacia is observed among those born with very low weight (<1500 g). The roots of this pathology can be found in (1) poor vascularization of white matter in premature infants and (2) prevalence of oligodendrocyte progenitors, which are particularly sensitive to ischaemia, reactive oxygen species and glutamate excitotoxicity. Thus, periods of even comparatively mild ischaemia result in profound damage to white matter and the demise of many oligodendrocyte progenitors. This, in turn, leads to defective myelination, with further defects in cerebral cortex development and impairment of pyramidal tracts, with subsequent neurological disorders, including cerebral palsy and cognitive defects.

10.5.3 Alzheimer's disease

Alzheimer's disease (AD), together with multi-infarct dementia, is the main cause of senile dementia. AD, named after Alois Alzheimer, who was the first to describe this pathology in 1907, is characterized by profound neuronal loss throughout the brain which rapidly compromises memory and results in severe impairment of cognitive functions. Histological hallmarks of AD are represented by the formation of deposits of β-amyloid protein (Aβ) in the walls of blood vessels, accumulation of Aβ plaques in the grey matter and intra-neuronal accumulation of abnormal tau-protein filaments in the form of neuronal tangles. AD is also characterized by prominent reactive astrogliosis and activation of microglia (incidentally, the involvement of glial cells in pathogenesis of AD was initially suggested by Alois

Alzheimer himself in 1910). In fact, AD plaques are formed by Aβ deposits, degenerating neurites, astroglial processes and activated microglial cells.

The specific role of astrocytes in the pathogenesis of AD began to be considered after it was discovered that astrocytes are natural scavengers of Aβ, and its particularly toxic truncated form Aβ42 (Aβ42 is a fragment of Aβ, which contains 42 amino acids and is the product of cleavage of amyloid precursor protein by beta- and gamma secretases). Astrocytes can detect and extend their processes towards deposits of Aβ, and then astrocytes are able to take up and degrade the Aβ. One of the possible (and recently discussed) scenarios of AD progression may be the following (Figure 10.7). At the very early stages of AD, neurones start to overproduce Aβ, which compromises their dendrites and leads to their degeneration and release of Aβ and other neuronal products; these activate astrocytes whose domains embrace the compromised neurone. Astrocytes begin to clear the neuronal debris and accumulate the Aβ. Remarkably, AD results in a selective increase of the neuronal type of nicotinic acetylcholine receptor (so-called α7nACHRs) in astroglial cells; incidentally, Aβ42 has a very high affinity for α7nACHRs, which probably explains the high vulnerability of cholinergic neurones to AD. It may well be that Aβ42 is accumulated by astrocytes together with α7nACHRs. Astrocytes eventually become overloaded with Aβ, which affects their function and results in decreased support of other neuronal processes within the astrocyte domain. This may initiate degeneration of the next neurone and trigger distant accumulation of Aβ. Importantly, astrocytes may even be instrumental in providing the route for Aβ neurotoxicity: *in vitro* experiments have shown that treatment of astroglial–neuronal co-cultures with Aβ results in the appearance of $[Ca^{2+}]_i$ oscillations in astrocytes, without any apparent $[Ca^{2+}]_i$ changes in neurones. Nonetheless, these astroglial oscillations led to neuronal death in ~24 hours; inhibition of glial $[Ca^{2+}]_i$ responses was neuroprotective. When the whole domain is thus degenerated, it undergoes lysis and the initial plaque is formed. Then, neighbouring astrocytes detect the extracellular Aβ deposit, become activated and send their processes towards the plaque, trying to clear the excess of Aβ. The repetition of this process eventually recruits increasing numbers of astrocytes and through them astrocytic domains with their neurones, which in turn leads to dissemination of the plaques. The latter in fact are polymorphic and may be formed either by lysis of neurones and astrocytes or by local death of astroglial cells only. The pathogenesis of AD also affects oligodendrocytes, whereby AD is associated with significant loss of myelin, which affects tracts connecting cortical areas.

The process of cell death and plaque formation triggers activation of microglia, which occurs both locally in the vicinity of the plaques and diffusely throughout the brain parenchyma. Activated microglia surround the plaques and participate in their formation. The actual role of microglia in AD progression remains unclear, as they may have both protective and deleterious effects. The initial suggestion that activated microglia may accumulate and remove Aβ fibrils, although observed *in vitro* in microglial cultures treated with Aβ, has not been confirmed *in vivo*.

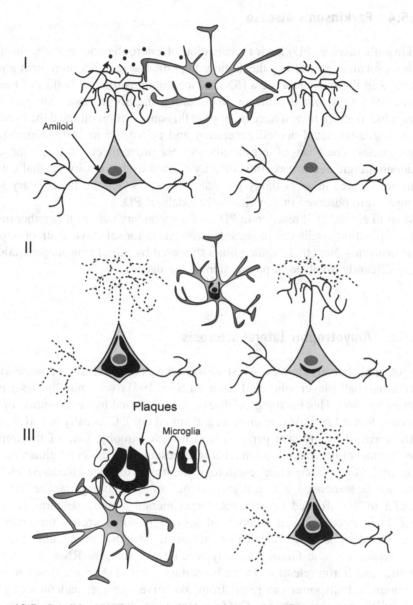

I

Amiloid

II

Plaques

III

Microglia

Figure 10.7 Possible role of astrocytes in the pathogenesis of Alzheimer's disease. In the first stage of the disease astrocytes detect β-amyloid, released by affected neurones, and withdraw their processes from both affected and neighbouring, intact, neurones. This leads to the second stage, when neurites lacking astroglial support begin to degenerate; the astrocyte by itself starts to accumulate β-amyloid. In the third stage neurones and astrocytes die and their debris attracts activated microglial cells and induces reactive astrogliosis. Reactive astrocytes, activated microglial cells and β-amyloid released from dead cells form the plaque. (Modified from Nagele RG, Wegiel J, Venkataraman V, Imaki H, Wang KC (2004) Contribution of glial cells to the development of amyloid plaques in Alzheimer's disease. *Neurobiol Aging* **25**, 663–74)

10.5.4   Parkinson's disease

Parkinson's disease (PD) leads to activation of microglia and reactive astrogliosis in the brain areas affected by the disease. In particular, a rather prominent gliosis is observed in the substantia nigra (SN), which contains the cell bodies of neurones forming the nigrostriatal pathway. Importantly, the SN neurones are particularly vulnerable to attack by activated microglia; this observation initiated the hypothesis of microglia-mediated neurodegeneration and cell death as instrumental for PD pathogenesis. The changes in astroglia are less pronounced, although the degree of dopaminergic neurone death is directly related to the density of glial cells: the neurones located in areas thinly populated by astrocytes die faster. Very similar changes were observed in experimental models of PD.

Most likely the glial reaction in PD is of a secondary nature: it is rather unlikely that malfunction of glia can be regarded as a cause for selective death of dopaminergic neurones. Nonetheless, the gliosis triggered by initial neurodegeneration can be significantly involved in progression of the disease.

10.5.5   Amyotrophic lateral sclerosis

Amyotrophic lateral sclerosis (ALS), also known as 'Lou Gehrig's disease' (named after a baseball player who died from ALS in 1941) was initially described by Charcot in 1869. This neurological disease is manifested by degeneration of motor neurones located in cortex, brain stem and spinal cord. Clinically the ALS appears in the form of progressive paralysis and muscle atrophy. One of the important determinants of neuronal death in ALS is represented by deficient glutamate clearance, and as a consequence, excitotoxic neuronal damage. Reduced glutamate clearance is associated with a disappearance of astroglial glutamate transporter EAAT2 in the affected brain areas. Experimental genetic deletion of EAAT2 (GLT-1) in mice led to a pronounced loss of motor neurones thus mimicking ALS. The disappearance of EAAT2 in human astroglia in sporadic ALS is the consequence of gene failure and may result from aberrant RNA splicing, exon skipping and intron retention. In the hereditary form of ALS the down-regulation of glutamate transporter can result from oxidative damage; patients carry mutations in a gene that encodes Cu/Zn superoxide dismutase (SOD1); the latter being an enzyme that converts superoxide radicals to hydrogen peroxide. Aberrant SOD1 results in an increased vulnerability of neurones and astrocytes to oxidative damage; furthermore it mediates (in an as yet unknown way) down-regulation of EAAT2 expression. In addition to deficient glutamate clearance, astrocytes may participate in neuronal damage through increased glutamate release: patients with ALS are reported to have increased levels of cyclooxygenase 2, which in turn produces prostaglandin E2; the latter is a potent activator of glutamate release from astrocytes.

10.6 Neuropathic pain

Peripheral neuropathic chronic pain is a severe and debilitating pathological condition which affects many millions of people. Neuropathic pain is a consequence of either neurotropic infections (most notably HIV) or injuries of peripheral nerves, which may occur following trauma, nerve compression or diabetes. The mechanisms of neuropathic pain are poorly understood and existing therapy is often ineffective. Very recently the role of glial cells, particularly microglia and to a lesser extent astroglia, as primary mediators of chronic pain, has begun to be considered and gained substantial experimental support. It is now firmly established that injury to peripheral nerve causes rapid and significant activation of microglia in the dorsal horn of the spinal cord on the side of the peripheral nerve entry (Figure 10.8). The activated microglial cells in spinal cord express pain related signalling molecules – P2X$_4$ purinoreceptors and p38 mitogen-activated protein kinase (p38 MAPK). The activation of P2X$_4$ receptors is necessary and sufficient to produce allodynia (pain arising from stimuli which are normally not painful), which is a very common symptom of chronic pain. Direct injection of P2X$_4$ stimulated microglia into rat spinal cord triggers allodynia; conversely, pharmacological inhibition of P2X$_4$ receptors reverses allodynia following experimental peripheral nerve injury. Similarly important is microglial p38 MAPK, which is rapidly activated following nerve injury, and pharmacological inhibition

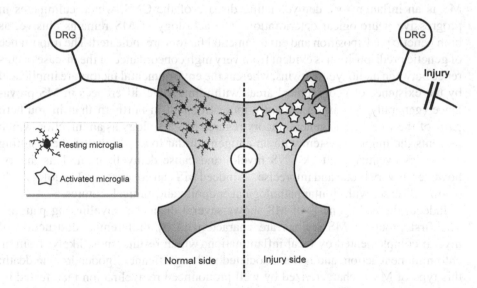

Figure 10.8 Activation of microglia as a mediator of neuropathic pain. Injury of peripheral nerves triggers activation of microglia in the ipsilateral side of the dorsal horn. This activation is mediated through P2X$_4$ ionotropic purinoreceptors and contributes to the development of chronic pain. (Modified from Tsuda M, Inoue K, Salter MW (2005) Neuropathic pain and spinal microglia: a big problem from molecules in 'small' glia. *Trends Neurosci* **28**, 101–107)

of p38 MAPK attenuates neuropathic pain symptoms. How microglia affect spinal cord sensory neurones and increase their excitability (which in turn underlies the enhanced firing discharges of these neurones and produces the sensation of pathological pain) remains unknown; it could be mediated by various neuroactive substances (such as ATP or proinflammatory cytokines) released by activated microglia, acting directly or as intermediate signals.

Spinal cord astrocytes also demonstrate signs of reactive gliosis following peripheral nerve injury. These astrocytes express some receptors related to pain; most notably vanilloid receptors type 1 (also known as capsaicin receptors; activated by obnoxious heat and chilli pepper) and cannabinoid receptors type 1. Peripheral nerve injury increases the synthesis of growth factors (e.g. FGF2) and cytokines in astroglial cells in the spinal cord. The precise role played by astrocytes in chronic pain remains to be uncovered.

10.7   Demyelinating diseases

10.7.1   Multiple sclerosis

Multiple sclerosis (MS) was recognized by the mid 19th century, and already in 1871 Hammond referred to it as a cerebrospinal sclerosis; it was Charcot who, in 1877, realized the role of disrupted myelin in the pathogenesis of this disease. MS is an inflammatory demyelinating disease of the CNS, which culminates in progressive neurological deterioration. The aetiology of MS remains elusive, as both genetic predisposition and environmental factors are indicated. The importance of genetic predisposition is evident from very high concordance of the disease occurrence between monozygotic twins, whereas the environmental factors are implicated by the existence of geographical areas with remarkable differences in MS prevalence (generally, MS is significantly more frequent in northern than in southern parts of the world). The general theory regards MS aetiology as an infection which presents the immune system with an antigen similar to CNS myelin; the resulting antibodies eventually attack CNS myelin and cause demyelination. This theory, however, is very broad and imprecise, as indeed MS can cover several aetiologically distinct diseases with similar pathological endpoint and clinical features.

Indeed, the pathogenesis of MS shows several distinct demyelinating patterns. The first group of MS lesions are characterized by preferential destruction of myelin complemented by local inflammation; which results, most likely, from an autoimmune reaction, and is not associated with significant oligodendrocyte death; this type of MS is characterized by well pronounced remyelination manifested by clinical remissions. The second type of MS progression is associated with oligodendrocyte death, which may happen either through apoptosis or necrosis. This form of MS progression is more violent, and patients with necrotic oligodendrocyte death are diagnosed with the so-called 'primary progressive' disease which does not show any relapses, and severe neurological deterioration. Moreover, the apoptotic death of oligodendrocytes has begun to be considered as the key step in initiation of MS pathological development, which may precede the autoimmune attack.

Importantly, however, in both types of disease pathogenesis, the areas of demyelination always show the signs of inflammatory processes and are rich in activated T lymphocytes. The latter can in fact cross the blood–brain barrier, and can attack the antigen-presenting tissue, which in the case of MS are myelin components or some parts of oligodendrocytes or both. At the same time, MS is accompanied with a degree of microglia activation; the activated microglia may be involved in regulating/shaping the immune response and somehow affecting the course of demyelination/oligodendrocyte death. Yet, the actual mechanisms which determine the progression of MS, and the role of different cellular elements in it, remains unresolved. Particularly interesting is the question of the initiation of oligodendroglial death, which can involve the Ca^{2+} toxic route; there are some indications that incubation of oligodendrocytes with antibodies to myelin–oligodendrocyte glycoprotein triggers $[Ca^{2+}]_i$ elevations and activation of intracellular kinases. Glutamate-mediated Ca^{2+} dependent excitotoxicity is also indicated in oligodendrocyte loss in MS.

10.7.2 Vanishing white matter disease

Vanishing white matter disease (VWM) is one of the most prevalent inherited childhood white-matter disorders. It was described in 1962 by Eicke. VWM is caused by mutations in any of the five genes encoding the subunits of eukaryotic translation initiation factor eIF2B, and is manifested by chronic progressive neurological deterioration with cerebellar ataxia and mild mental decline. The disease is usually revealed at an early age of two to six years, and most of the patients die within several years after diagnosis.

VWM disease stems from a severe deterioration of white matter, which shows myelin loss, abnormal formation of myelin sheaths, vacuolation; the white matter degenerates and appears cystic; cavities are often observed. Around these cavities a pronounced loss of oligodendrocytes is detected; many oligodendrocytes also have an abnormal morphological appearance. The astrocytes are dysmorphic with blunt broad processes rather than their typical delicate arborizations.

There is no specific treatment for VWM.

10.8 Infectious diseases

10.8.1 Bacterial and viral infections

Bacterial and viral infections of brain parenchyma invariably trigger reactive astrogliosis and activation of microglia; these processes may be local (e.g. in the case of brain abscesses) or diffuse (e.g. upon encephalitis). Reactive astrogliosis and activation of microglia are components of the brain's defence reactions, and in fact their success very much determines the outcome of infection.

Glial reactions can be acute (e.g. in the case of acute meningitis or encephalitis) or chronic (e.g. upon infections evoked by *Toxoplasma gondii*, which persists in neurones). Sometimes, glial reactions can be the first step in pathogenesis of the disease, which often happens upon viral infections such as HIV (which is discussed in detail below) or Borna virus. In the latter case, reactive astrogliosis occurs prior to the onset of encephalitis, and astrocytes begin to produce many inflammatory proteins, including interferon-γ-inducible protein and inflammatory protein-10, which are important for further development of the disease. It is quite possible that astrocytes become infected by Borna viruses early in the progression of the disease; and the virus-stimulated secretion of chemokines and cytokines as well as inflammatory proteins is important for attraction of invading T lymphocytes, able to cope with viral infection. In particular, astroglial synthesis and release of inflammatory protein-10 is a possible general mechanism of astroglial reaction to viruses, as similar changes were observed during CNS infections with hepatitis virus, adenovirus and lymphocytic choriomeningitis virus; inflammatory protein-10 also has a direct antiviral effect against herpes simplex virus.

Bacterial infections usually affect the subarachnoid space, and result in meningitis without affecting the brain parenchyma, and therefore, as a rule, glial reactions are relatively mild. Bacterial meningitis results in activation of numerous immunological responses including activation of the complement system and release of C3a and C5a anaphylatoxins. The reactive glial cells are concentrated in brain layers located closely to the meninges, and may participate in local defensive and immune reactions. Certain bacterial infections, such as infections with grampositive *Streptococcus pneumoniae* may trigger over-activation of microglia (and indeed the pneumococcal cell walls are extremely efficient microglia activators), which may in turn be involved in diffuse brain damage; this particular role of activated microglia may be a reason for the exceptionally high mortality and treatment resistance of gram-positive brain infections.

10.8.2   Human immunodeficiency virus (HIV) infection

Brain damage is a frequent outcome of acquired immunodeficiency syndrome (AIDS), the pathology manifesting in a form of *HIV-encephalitis* (*HIVE*). The latter progresses through cognitive impairments, psychomotor abnormalities, including ataxia, towards severe *HIV-associated dementia* (*HAD*). In addition to HAD, AIDS also produces HIV-related sensory neuropathies. The combined prevalence of HIV-associated dementia and sensory neuropathies can reach up to 50 per cent in all patients.

Microglia and perivascular macrophages are the principal target for HIV infection of the brain; the virus essentially cannot infect neurones. To infect the cells the HIV uses surface receptors for chemokines (e.g. CD4 or CCR5), which, in the brain parenchyma are mostly associated with microglia. The virus can invade the brain very soon after infection, yet at the latent stages it does not result in any productive infection. There are some indications that during this latent stage, the virus can survive in the brain within the microglial cells, the latter serving as a reservoir (so-called Trojan horse) for HIV, which can reinfect the periphery; this is particularly important in the targeting of antiviral drug therapies. This long-lasting presence of HIV in the brain parenchyma may explain the appearance of CNS-specific strain variances. Viral HAD commences only after onset of AIDS, and then the production of virus in the CNS is very significant.

Histopathologically, HAD is manifested by prominent neuronal death (usually though the apoptotic pathway), the neuronal demise being most prominent in the basal ganglia. The histological hallmark of HIVE/HAD is the appearance of *multinucleated giant cells*, which represent fused infected microglia/macrophages. Astroglial cells show fewer changes; in fact astrocytes (which also contain surface chemokine receptors) can be readily infected by HIV *in vitro*; however their infection in the *in vivo* brain is much less documented.

The neurotoxicity in HIVE results from two principal sources: from viral products and from activated microglia/macrophages. The cytotoxic viral components are glycoprotein 120 (gp120 assists virus binding to plasmalemmal receptors and entry into the cell), *tat* protein, which acts as a viral transactivator, and Vpr protein. Gp120 kills neurones both *in vitro* (after being added to culture media) and *in vivo* (when gp120 was delivered by intra-hippocampal injection). Direct induction of astroglial expression of gp120 in transgenic mice resulted in the development of brain damage similar to HIVE. The actual neurotoxic action of gp120 is mediated through disruption of neuronal Ca^{2+} homeostasis and Ca^{2+} excitotoxicity. Gp120 can cause both sustained Ca^{2+} entry and massive Ca^{2+} release from the ER stores; the combination of the two causes Ca^{2+} overload and cell death. *Tat* protein also induces neuronal apoptosis; the latter can be initiated through Ca^{2+} dyshomeostasis. *Tat* protein was reported to induce substantial increases in neuronal $[Ca^{2+}]_i$ through activation of NMDA receptors; these $[Ca^{2+}]_i$ elevations led to neuronal death; both Ca^{2+} increase and cell demise can be prevented by NMDA receptor blockers. *Tat* is also able to trigger Ca^{2+} signals in microglia through CCR3 chemokine receptors; these Ca^{2+} signals may assist in spreading the microglial activation. Finally, *tat* may also stimulate reactive astrogliosis. The Vpr protein triggers apoptotic neuronal death *in vitro* through yet unknown mechanisms.

The second important source of neuronal death is associated with neurotoxic agents released by activated microglia, which in the case of HIVE fully realizes its pathological potential. In fact the relative HIV production in the brain is not dramatic; it is much less, for example, than production of other neurotropic viruses such as herpes simplex or arboviruses. Therefore, the activated microglia and macrophages may be the leading players in mediating neuronal cell death in HIVE/HAD.

10.9   Peripheral neuropathies

10.9.1   Hereditary neuropathies

There are several hereditary neuropathies, associated with mutation of genes encoding either myelin or specific Schwann cell proteins. These genetic pathologies of Schwann cells include the Charcot-Marie-Tooth disease (CMT), hereditary neuropathy with liability to pressure palsies (HNPP), Roussy–Levy syndrome and congenital hypomyelinating neuropathy (CHN).

Charcot-Marie-Tooth disease, also known as peroneal muscular atrophy, covers several disorders characterized by progressive deterioration of peripheral innervation. At least some of the incidences of CMT disease are the autosomal-recessive demyelinating neuropathy, which is caused by transmission of mutated gene(s), encoding the so-called 'ganglioside-induced differentiation-associated protein 1' (or GDAP1), which is believed to be involved in permanent bridging of Schwann cells and axons. Other variants of CMT are associated with duplication of chromosome 17. The disease is characterized by rapidly developing demyelination and axonal degradation, which trigger paralysis and early death. Additionally, some versions of CMT result from mutations in connexin 32, the main gap junctional protein in the PNS. Roussy–Levy syndrome is a variant of CMT, which is manifested by tremor and weakness in upper limbs, sensory loss and ataxia; it may arise from the mutation of the gene encoding P0, which is involved in adhesion of compact myelin (see Chapter 8), or from chromosomal disorders, e.g. particle duplication of chromosome 17.

Hereditary neuropathy with liability to pressure palsies results from deletion of point mutation in the same chromosome 17, which affect the gene encoding PMP22, which stabilizes the myelin sheath. HNPP pathology stems from dysmyelination, as numerous redundant layers, loops or folds of myelin (known as tomaculae) are produced. This altered myelin production eventually results in prominent axonal death. Finally, congenital hypomyelinating neuropathy can be caused by various mutations, which affect the production of myelin. In particular CHN can be associated with mutations in the gene encoding periaxin, which is important for Schwann cell–axonal interactions. Alternatively hypomyelination syndromes can result from mutations in dystrophin gene.

10.9.2   Acquired inflammatory neuropathies

Acquired peripheral neuropathies are broadly classified into acute and chronic inflammatory demyelinating neuropathies (AIDP and CIDP, respectively). Clinical forms of these neuropathies are many, and all of them proceed with sensory abnormalities or motor weaknesses, or a combination of both. Pathogenetically inflammatory neuropathies belong to autoimmune diseases; the actual neuropathy usually follows viral infection; the latter triggers an immune response, which turns into an autoimmune reaction aimed at myelin or protein components of Schwann cells. Important roles are played by antibodies against viral oligosaccharide components, which are, incidentally, identical to gangliosides (GM1 or GD1a) of the peripheral nerve; as a result, antibodies produced against viruses attack the body's own tissue. In addition, certain infections may produce antibodies against myelin proteins, most frequently against protein PMP22.

The autoreactive T cells, bearing the autoantibodies, migrate towards the peripheral nerve, and (by release of cytokines and chemokines) recruit macrophages, which attack both Schwann cells and myelin sheaths. Initially, macrophages form infiltrations within the peripheral nerve, and destroy the myelin; subsequently, they phagocytose the remnants of the glial cells and demyelinated axons.

10.9.3 Diabetic neuropathies

Diabetic neuropathies are the most frequent complications of diabetes mellitus, which affect ~50 per cent of all patients. Clinically, the sensory neuropathies dominate; motor weakness develops rather rarely. The primary cause of nerve damage is associated with blood glucose levels; aggressive glycaemic control substantially reduces the prevalence of neuropathies. The primary target of the impaired glucose homeostasis is, however, debatable. Traditionally, the leading aetiological factor was associated with abnormalities in neurovascular circulation, which indeed suffers remarkably. According to these theories, the nerve damage was a direct consequence of poor circulation, ischaemia and oxidative injury. Yet, in many cases neuropathies develop without any obvious degradation in neurocirculation. An alternative theory stresses the pathogenetic importance of Schwann cells, which are particularly sensitive to hyperglycaemia; the latter damage glial cells mostly through oxidative stress. Indeed, diabetes is associated with significant morphological abnormalities of Schwann cells and high incidence of their apoptotic death. The obvious consequence of Schwann cells demise is demyelination and reduced nerve conductance velocity, which is the most common symptom of diabetic neuropathy.

10.9.4 Leprosy

Leprosy is the primary infectious disease of Schwann cells. The infectious agent, *Mycobacterium leprae*, specifically invades the Schwann cells, where it multiplies with impunity, being protected by organism-specific host immunity. The infected Schwann cells eventually die, thus triggering powerful immune reactions, which in turn destroy myelin and kill the axons, hence producing profound nerve damage. This nerve damage defines the clinical signature of the disease, which progresses as an acute neuropathy, resulting initially in anaesthetic skin patches, and later in trophic and motor abnormalities. The pathogenic involvement of autoimmune components is important for therapeutic strategy, which currently relies on a combination of immunodepression and anti-mycobacterial therapy.

10.10 Psychiatric diseases

10.10.1 Epilepsy

Epilepsy results from abnormal synchrony in the neuronal networks, when many nerve cells start to fire simultaneously. These discharges can be visualized on the EEG, which reveals cortical spikes and sharp waves. The cellular substrate of epilepsy is a slow depolarization of neurones, which occurs without any apparent provocation and develops synchronously in virtually all nerve cells within the epileptic foci. This slow neuronal depolarization is known as *paroxysmal depolarization shift*, PDS.

The PDS results from large excitatory postsynaptic potentials, which develop slower than normal EPSPs, triggered by electrical excitation of incoming synaptic terminals; usually the PDS lasts from 50 to 200 ms. The synaptic potential underlying the PDS is mediated by glutamate receptors of AMPA and NMDA types, and is caused by simultaneous glutamate release around many neurones comprising epileptic foci. When the PDS fails to terminate, the prolonged synchronous depolarization of many neurones results in seizures, which are the hallmarks of epilepsy.

Astrocytes begin to be involved in pathogenesis of epilepsy at very early stages of the disease; they become reactive, they are hypertrophied, change their shape and increase in number and this reactive astrogliosis occurs before any neurodegenerative changes and even before the appearance of fully developed seizures. Physiologically, neuronal PSD and seizures lead to depolarization of astrocytes surrounding the epileptic zone.

Very recently it has become apparent that PSD can still develop in conditions of synaptic isolation – i.e. when neuronal firing is completely blocked by tetrodotoxin, which effectively poisons Na^+ channels. Moreover, it was also shown that local stimulation of astroglial $[Ca^{2+}]_i$ signals in brain slices prepared from hippocampus can trigger release of glutamate, which in turn initiates PSD and epileptiform discharges in neighbouring neurones. Moreover, glial $[Ca^{2+}]_i$ waves always preceded spontaneous PSD in the brains of animals experimentally made epileptic.

This new knowledge about the role of astrocytes in producing neuronal epileptiform activity will considerably change our understanding of epilepsy pathogenesis. In fact, the introduction of astrocytes into the epileptic circuit (Figure 10.9) can be instrumental in describing the most enigmatic property of the epileptic brain – i.e. the precise synchronization between many neurones. This synchronization may result, for example, from abnormal glutamate release from an individual astrocyte, which can reach up to 100 000 synapses within the astroglial domain,

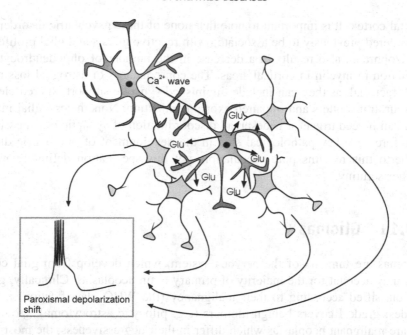

Figure 10.9 Astroglia and epileptic seizures. Astroglial calcium waves may trigger synchronous release of glutamate, which in turn may act simultaneously on many neurones and trigger the specific depolarization, the paroxysmal depolarization shift, considered to be the electrical correlate of epileptic seizure

virtually simultaneously. Furthermore, several astroglial cells can work as a single unit, being synchronized through gap junctions, and then the number of neurones affected by one simultaneous glutamate discharge can be much greater. These new insights into the pathology of epilepsy may also considerably modify the quest for new therapeutic strategies, as astroglial cells may well be the primary target. Incidentally, several anti-epileptic drugs, including valproate, gabapentin and phenytoin, are able to inhibit astroglial Ca^{2+} signalling, which may, at least in part, account for their anticonvulsant potency.

10.10.2 Schizophrenia, bipolar disorder and major depressive disorder

All three major psychiatric disorders, schizophrenia, bipolar disorder (BP) and major depressive disorder (MDD) affect brain cytoarchitecture. Along with numerous histopathological signals of neuronal malfunction (e.g. reduction in neuronal size, dendritic length and dendritic spines density), these diseases also affect glial cells. There are some indications for loss of astrocytes and GFAP expression in schizophrenia, BP and MDD. In BP and MDD, significant decreases in the numbers and volume of astroglial cells were detected in prefrontal and orbital cortex. It is important to note that none of these psychiatric disorders were considered previously to be associated with reactive gliosis and glial proliferation. Schizophrenia also results in a decrease in the number of oligodendrocytes and reduction in myelin in cortical areas. The consequences of astroglial loss may be multifactorial, as they can include diminished synaptic support, altered clearance of neurotransmitters and impaired axonal conduction. Nonetheless, glial malfunction can indeed trigger a widespread discoordination of synaptic transmission and therefore be a key pathological step in the development of psychiatric diseases. Hitherto this remains pure speculation, yet this speculation definitely warrants further scrutiny.

10.11 Gliomas

Gliomas are tumours of the nervous system, which develop from glial cells; in fact they account for the majority of primary brain neoplasias. Clinically, gliomas are classified according to their malignancy (the WHO classification) into four grades: grade I covers benign tumours (e.g. pilocytic astrocytoma), groups II to IV are malignant neoplasias which differ in their aggressiveness; the most violent is glioblastoma, which belongs to group IV. Histopathologically, the gliomas are divided into *astrocytomas*, *oligodendrocytomas* and *glioblastomas*; although this division mostly relates to morphological similarity of tumour cell to the respective types of macroglia; the exact origin of the cancerous 'stem' cell cannot be revealed with much precision.

  Biologically, the gliomas are very different from other neoplasias, as they express several systems which adapt them to malignant growth within the CNS environment. The main property of the latter is the lack of free space into which the tumour can grow, and the existence of firm boundaries (skull for the brain and vertebrae for spinal cord) which present additional restraints for neoplasia expansion. The second complication of the CNS architecture, from the point of view of cancerous growth, is a very complicated structure of parenchyma, formed by extremely narrow and low volume clefts; these prevent free dissemination of malignant cells through the tissue, which is so characteristic for tumour expansion in non-brain organs. Therefore, in order to grow gliomas must clear the space by actively eliminating the surrounding healthy cells, and actively propagate neoplasmic cells though the brain matter.

  Malignant gliomas produce the room for their expansion by actively killing neurones in their vicinity. This is achieved by secretion of high amounts of glutamate, which in turn triggers excitotoxic, NMDA- and $[Ca^{2+}]_i$-dependent neuronal death. This glutamate-induced neuronal death also results in seizures, which often accompany malignant gliomas. The amount of glutamate synthesized and released by glioma cells is truly impressive: e.g. cultured glioma cells can increase glutamate concentration in their media from 1 μM to 100 μM within 5–6 hours. Release of glutamate is mediated through an electroneutral amino acid transporter

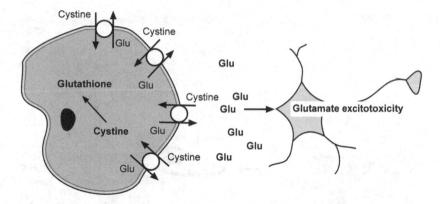

Figure 10.10 Glioma induced neuronal death. Glioma cells express high density of gluta-mate/cystine transporter; glutamate released by this transporter triggers excitotoxic neuronal death, thus clearing space for glioma invasion

which exchanges cystine for glutamate; this transporter is specifically expressed only in glioma cells (Figure 10.10). Glutamate excitotoxicity is critical for glioma expansion; inhibition of the cystine/glutamate transporter (which can be blocked by 4-carboxyphenylglycine) has been shown to significantly retard their growth. Cystine brought into the glioma cells is converted into glutathione, which increases resistance of tumour cells to oxidative stress.

The second important peculiarity of gliomas is represented by their active prop-agation through the nervous tissue. Glioma cells are able to travel through the brain, e.g. they easily migrate from one hemisphere to another. As a consequence, gliomas almost invariably disseminate through the whole brain. The mechanisms of glioma cell migration are several. First, they express a number of metallo-proteinases, which assist in breaking down the extracellular matrix, and produce migrating tunnels. Second, glioma cells are able to undergo substantial shrinkage, which helps them to attain an elongated shape and thus penetrate into narrow interstitial compartments. This loss of glioma cell volume is supported by several families of Cl^- channels, which are activated by voltage or changes in osmolarity; in addition, glioma cells express Cl^- permeable GABA receptors. Glioma cells have a high concentration of cytoplasmic Cl^-, which sets the Cl^- reversal poten-tial at levels more positive than the resting potential (–40 mV); activation of Cl^- channels therefore leads to Cl^- efflux, which in turn drives water out of the cell, therefore reducing its volume (Figure 10.11). Inhibition of Cl^- channels arrests the motility of glioma cells. Finally, glioma migration is also driven by cytosolic Ca^{2+} oscillations, which results from the activation of Ca^{2+}-permeable AMPA receptors. Inhibition of Ca^{2+} permeability of AMPA receptors suppresses glioma dissemina-tion and limits the tumour growth. All in all, glioma cells utilize several purely neural mechanisms to expand within the CNS; these mechanisms also render high malignancy and rapid clinical progression of glial-derived tumours.

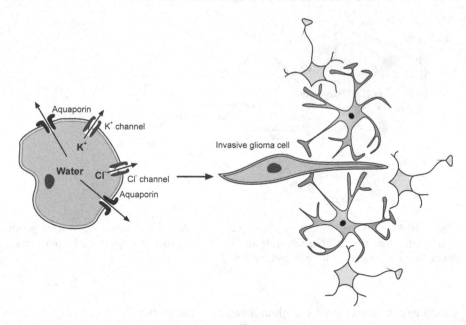

Figure 10.11 Chloride and potassium channels assist glioma cell shrinkage; decrease in glioma cell volume greatly facilitates their invasive capabilities. To shrink, glioma cells release K$^+$ and Cl$^-$ through ion channels, which induce water to leave the cells through aquaporins. The maintenance of K$^+$ and Cl$^-$ concentration in glioma is accomplished by the activity of the NKCC Cl$^-$ transporter and the Na$^+$–K$^+$ ATPase. (Modified from McFerrin MB, Sontheimer H (2006) A role for ion channels in glioma cell invasion. *Neuron Glia Biol* **2**, 39–49)

10.11.1   Glial complications of glioma therapy

Irradiation therapy of gliomas often results in cognitive and memory decline of a yet undiscovered nature. One of the current hypotheses highlights the role of activated hippocampal microglia, which may interfere with neurogenesis. Indeed it was found that irradiation of the brain causes activation of microglia and inhibition of neurogenesis; a very similar result was obtained after intra-hippocampal injections of LPS, which is a powerful microglial activator. Neurogenesis can be restored and activation of microglia placated by anti-inflammatory drugs such as indomethacin, or by inhibitors of microglial activation such as minocycline.

Conclusions

Although the glia was discovered before neurones, its importance in the function of the nervous system was neglected for a long time. The tide has turned, however, during the last twenty years, and a multitude of seminal discoveries have been made. All in all general neurobiology reluctantly agreed that glial cells are as important as neurones for brain function and glia cannot be bluntly disregarded anymore. This has changed our perception of how the brain is organized, and how the development, life and death of neural circuits are controlled. Indeed, astrocytes appear to be omnipotent neural progenitors, and the same astrocytes mostly control synaptogenesis, define microarchitecture of the brain, and form neuronal–glial–vascular units. In fact it is astrocytes which brunt the all-important task of integrating various cells and structures of the brain into individual units, simultaneously connecting these units into the functional entity. Astrocytes are capable of sensing and releasing transmitter, thus being fully involved in ongoing brain chemical transmission, yet in addition the astroglial syncytium, connected through gap junction communication pathways, allows an alternative and sophisticated intercellular communication route, which permits direct translocation of ions, metabolic factors and second messengers. The resulting potential for parallel processing and integration is significant and might easily be larger, but also fuzzier, than the binary coded electrical communication within the neuronal networks. In a way, the neuronal networks may be seen as highly specialized elements of rapid delivery of information, whereas astroglial cells may represent the true substrate (or 'substance', as Virchow would have called it) for information processing, integration and storage. Indeed, the number of glia, both in absolute terms and relative to the number of neurones, increases dramatically on the phylogenetic scale, and the complexity of glial cells is the greatest in the human brain, where the intelligence also dwells.

The extremely elaborated panglial syncytium is a true neural reticulum, which, at least in numerical terms prevails over discreet neuronal networks; although both internally connected glial syncytium and discreet neuronal networks peacefully coexist within the brain. Shall we anticipate even more exciting discoveries which eventually can challenge the role of neurones as sole origins of intellect and cognition? Can the neuronal doctrine withstand the challenge from glial cells? This is the future, which holds a definite answer to this question.

Glial Neurobiology: A Textbook   Alexei Verkhratsky and Arthur Butt
© 2007 John Wiley & Sons, Ltd   ISBN 978-0-470-01564-3 (HB); 978-0-470-51740-6 (PB)

Recommended literature

Handbooks and monographs

Kettenmann H, Ransom BR (1985) *Neuroglia.* Oxford University Press, 1st edition.
Kettenmann H, Ransom BR (2005) *Neuroglia.* Oxford University Press 2nd edition.

Initial discoveries (Chapter 1)

First definition of glia as an integrative part of brain parenchyma

Virchow R (1846) Über das granulierte Ansehen der Wandungen der Gehirnventrikel. *Allg Z Psychiatrie* **3**, 242–250.
Virchow R (1858) *Die Cellularpathologie in ihrer Begründung auf physiologische and pathologische Gewebelehre.* Verlag von August Hirschfeld, Berlin.

Early works on morphology of glia

Andriezen L (1893) The neuroglia elements in the human brain. *BMJ* **29**, 227–230.
Golgi C (1903) *Opera Omnia* (Vol. I–III). Hoepli Editore, Milano.
Ramón y Cajal S (1897–1904); trans. (1995) *Histology of the Nervous System of Man and Vertebrates.* Oxford University Press, Oxford.
Retzius GM (1881–1921) *Biologische Untersuchungen*, Vol. 1–6. Samson and Wallin, Stockholm.

First indication about functional connection between neurones and blood vessels

Golgi C (1871) Contribuzione alla fine anatomia degli organi centrali del sistema nervoso. *Rivista Clinica di Bologna* (in French).

First theory of active neuronal–glial interactions

Schleich CL (1894) *Schmerzlose Operationen. Oertliche Betäubung mit indiffrenten Flüssigkeiten.* Julius Springer, Berlin.

First electrophysiological recordings from glial cells

Kuffler SW, Potter DD (1964) Glia in the leech central nervous system: Physiological properties and neuron–glia relationship. *J Neurophysiol* **27**, 290–320.
Orkand RK, Nicholls JG, Kuffler SW (1966) Effect of nerve impulses on the membrane potential of glial cells in the central nervous system of amphibia. *J Neurophysiol* **29**, 788–806.
Verkhratsky A (2006) Patching the glia reveals the functional organisation of the brain. *Pflugers Arch* **453**, 411–420.

Glial Neurobiology: A Textbook   Alexei Verkhratsky and Arthur Butt
© 2007 John Wiley & Sons, Ltd   ISBN 978-0-470-01564-3 (HB); 978-0-470-51740-6 (PB)

Patch-clamp and calcium indicator techniques

Hamill OP, Marty A, Neher E, Sakmann B, Sigworth FJ (1981) Improved patch-clamp techniques for high-resolution current recording from cells and cell-free membrane patches. *Pflugers Arch* **391**, 85–100.

Tsien RY (1980) New calcium indicators and buffers with high selectivity against magnesium and protons: design, synthesis, and properties of prototype structures. *Biochemistry* **19**, 2396–2404.

Verkhratsky A, Krishtal OA, Petersen OH (2006) From Galvani to patch clamp: the development of electrophysiology. *Pflugers Arch* **453**, 233–247.

First discovery of functional neurotransmitter receptors in glia

Bowman CL, Kimelberg HK (1984) Excitatory amino acids directly depolarize rat brain astrocytes in primary culture. *Nature* **311**, 656–659.

Kettenmann H, Backus KH, Schachner M (1984) Aspartate, glutamate and gamma-aminobutyric acid depolarize cultured astrocytes. *Neurosci Lett* **52**, 25–29.

Kettenmann H, Gilbert P, Schachner M (1984) Depolarization of cultured oligodendrocytes by glutamate and GABA. *Neurosci Lett* **47**, 271–276.

Signalling in the nervous system (Chapter 2)

Volume and wiring transmission

Agnati LF, Zoli M, Stromberg I, Fuxe K (1995) Intercellular communication in the brain: wiring versus volume transmission. *Neuroscience* **69**, 711–726.

Bloom FE (2000) Integration of wiring transmission and volume transmission. *Prog Brain Res* **125**, 21–26.

Magistretti PJ, Pellerin L (2000) The astrocyte-mediated coupling between synaptic activity and energy metabolism operates through volume transmission. *Prog Brain Res* **125**, 229–240.

Sykova E (2005) Glia and volume transmission during physiological and pathological states. *J Neural Transm* **112**, 137–147.

Zoli M, Torri C, Ferrari R, Jansson A, Zini I, Fuxe K, Agnati LF (1998) The emergence of the volume transmission concept. *Brain Res Rev* **26**,136–147.

Intracellular signalling

Bigge CF (1999) Ionotropic glutamate receptors. *Curr Opin Chem Biol* **3**, 441–447.

Burnstock G (1972) Purinergic nerves. *Pharmacol Rev* **24**, 509–581.

Burnstock G (2006) Historical review: ATP as a neurotransmitter. *Trends Pharmacol Sci* **27**, 166–176.

Egan TM, Samways DS, Li Z (2006) Biophysics of P2X receptors. *Pflugers Arch* **452**, 501–512.

Hollmann M, Heinemann S (1994) Cloned glutamate receptors. *Annu Rev Neurosci* **17**, 31–108.

Hussl S, Boehm S (2006) Functions of neuronal P2Y receptors. *Pflugers Arch* **452**, 538–551.

Nakanishi S (1994) Metabotropic glutamate receptors: synaptic transmission, modulation, and plasticity. *Neuron* **13**, 1031–1037.

Nakanishi S, Nakajima Y, Masu M, Ueda Y, Nakahara K, Watanabe D, Yamaguchi S, Kawabata S, Okada M (1998) Glutamate receptors: brain function and signal transduction. *Brain Res Rev* **26**, 230–235.

North RA, Verkhratsky A (2006) Purinergic transmission in the central nervous system. *Pflugers Arch* **452**, 479–485.

Pin JP, Acher F (2002) The metabotropic glutamate receptors: structure, activation mechanism and pharmacology. *Curr Drug Targets CNS Neurol Disord* **1**, 297–317.

Schofield PR, Shivers BD, Seeburg PH (1990) The role of receptor subtype diversity in the CNS. *Trends Neurosci* **13**, 8–11.

Wisden W, Seeburg PH (1992) GABAA receptor channels: from subunits to functional entities. *Curr Opin Neurobiol* **2**, 263–269.

Wisden W, Seeburg PH (1993) Mammalian ionotropic glutamate receptors. *Curr Opin Neurobiol* **3**, 291–298.

Morphology of glia (Chapter 3)

Bushong EA, Martone ME, Jones YZ, Ellisman MH (2002) Protoplasmic astrocytes in CA1 stratum radiatum occupy separate anatomical domains. *J Neurosci* **22**, 183–192.

Nedergaard M, Ransom B, Goldman SA (2003) New roles for astrocytes: redefining the functional architecture of the brain. *Trends Neurosci* **26**, 523–530.

Ogata K, Kosaka T (2002) Structural and quantitative analysis of astrocytes in the mouse hippocampus. *Neuroscience* **113**, 221–233.

Glial development (Chapter 4)

Phylogeny of glia and evolutionary specificity of glial cells in human brain

Colombo JA, Reisin HD (2004) Interlaminar astroglia of the cerebral cortex: a marker of the primate brain. *Brain Res* **1006**, 126–131.

Oberheim NA, Wang X, Goldman S, Nedergaard M (2006) Astrocytic complexity distinguishes the human brain. *Trends Neurosci* **29**, 547–553.

Sherwood CC, Stimpson CD, Raghanti MA, Wildman DE, Uddin M, Grossman LI, Goodman M, Redmond JC, Bonar CJ, Erwin JM, Hof PR (2006) Evolution of increased glia–neuron ratios in the human frontal cortex. *Proc Natl Acad Sci U S A* **103**, 13606–13611.

Astrocytes in the brain of Albert Einstein

Colombo JA, Reisin HD, Miguel-Hidalgo JJ, Rajkowska G (2006) Cerebral cortex astroglia and the brain of a genius: a propos of A. Einstein's. *Brain Res Rev* **52**, 257–263.

Astrocytes as brain stem cells

Goldman S (2003) Glia as neural progenitor cells. *Trends Neurosci* **26**, 590–596.

Götz M, Barde YA (2005) Radial glial cells defined and major intermediates between embryonic stem cells and CNS neurons *Neuron* **46**, 369–372.

Horner PJ, Palmer TD (2003) New roles for astrocytes: the nightlife of an 'astrocyte'. La vida loca! *Trends Neurosci* **26**, 597–603.

Mori T, Buffo A, Götz M (2005) The novel roles of glial cells revisited: The contribution of radial glia and astrocytes to neurogenesis. *Current Topics Dev Biol* **69**, 67–99.

Glial physiology (Chapter 5)

Ion channels and neurotransmitter receptors

Barres BA, Chun LL, Corey DP (1988) Ion channel expression by white matter glia: I. Type 2 astrocytes and oligodendrocytes. *Glia* **1**, 10–30.

Barres BA, Koroshetz WJ, Swartz KJ, Chun LL, Corey DP (1990) Ion channel expression by white matter glia: the O-2A glial progenitor cell. *Neuron* **4**, 507–524.

Berger T, Schnitzer J, Orkand PM, Kettenmann H (1992) Sodium and calcium currents in glial cells of the mouse corpus callosum slice. *Eur J Neurosci* **4**, 1271–1284.

Fields RD, Burnstock G (2006) Purinergic signalling in neuron–glia interactions. *Nat Rev Neurosci* **7**, 423–436.

Karadottir R, Cavelier P, Bergersen LH, Attwell D (2005) NMDA receptors are expressed in oligodendrocytes and activated in ischaemia. *Nature* **438**, 1162–1166.

Lipton SA (2006) NMDA receptors, glial cells, and clinical medicine. *Neuron* **50**, 9–11.

MacVicar BA. (1984) Voltage-dependent calcium channels in glial cells. *Science* **226**, 1345–1347.

Seifert G, Steinhauser C (2001) Ionotropic glutamate receptors in astrocytes. *Prog Brain Res* **132**, 287–299.

Steinhauser C, Gallo V (1996) News on glutamate receptors in glial cells. *Trends Neurosci* **19**, 339–345.

Verkhratsky A, Kirchoff F (2007) NMDA receptors in glia. *Neuroscientist* **3**, 1–10

Verkhratsky A, Steinhauser C (2000) Ion channels in glial cells. *Brain Res Rev* **32**, 380–412.

Gap junctions, connexins and hemichannels
Bennett MV, Contreras JE, Bukauskas FF, Saez JC (2003) New roles for astrocytes: gap junction hemichannels have something to communicate. *Trends Neurosci* **26**, 610–617.

Dermietzel R (1998) Gap junction wiring: a 'new' principle in cell-to-cell communication in the nervous system? *Brain Res Rev* **26**, 176–83.

Evans WH, De Vuyst E, Leybaert L (2006) The gap junction cellular internet: connexin hemichannels enter the signalling limelight. *Biochem J* **397**, 1–14.

Nagy JI, Rash JE (2000) Connexins and gap junctions of astrocytes and oligodendrocytes in the CNS. *Brain Res Rev* **32**, 29–44.

Saez JC, Retamal MA, Basilio D, Bukauskas FF, Bennett MV (2005) Connexin-based gap junction hemichannels: gating mechanisms. *Biochim Biophys Acta* **1711**, 215–224.

Sosinsky GE, Nicholson BJ (2005) Structural organization of gap junction channels. *Biochim Biophys Acta* **1711**, 99–125.

Calcium signals and calcium waves
Cornell-Bell AH, Finkbeiner SM, Cooper MS, Smith SJ (1990) Glutamate induces calcium waves in cultured astrocytes: long-range glial signaling. *Science* **247**, 470–473.

Newman EA, Zahs KR (1997) Calcium waves in retinal glial cells. *Science* **275**, 844–847.

Scemes E, Giaume C (2006) Astrocyte calcium waves: what they are and what they do. *Glia* **54**, 716–725.

Verkhratsky A, Orkand RK, Kettenmann H (1998) Glial calcium: homeostasis and signaling function. *Physiol Rev* **78**, 99–141.

Verkhratsky A (2006) Calcium ions and integration in neural circuits. *Acta Physiol (Oxf)* **187**, 357–369.

Vesicular release of neurotransmitters
Bezzi P, Domercq M, Brambilla L, Galli R, Schols D, De Clercq E, Vescovi A, Bagetta G, Kollias G, Meldolesi J, Volterra A (2001) CXCR4-activated astrocyte glutamate release via TNFalpha: amplification by microglia triggers neurotoxicity. *Nat Neurosci* **4**, 702–710.

Bezzi P, Gundersen V, Galbete JL, Seifert G, Steinhauser C, Pilati E, Volterra A (2004) Astrocytes contain a vesicular compartment that is competent for regulated exocytosis of glutamate. *Nat Neurosci* **7**, 613–620.

Parpura V, Haydon PG (2000) Physiological astrocytic calcium levels stimulate glutamate release to modulate adjacent neurons. *Proc Natl Acad Sci U S A* **97**, 8629–8634.

Zhang Q, Fukuda M, Van Bockstaele E, Pascual O, Haydon PG (2004) Synaptotagmin IV regulates glial glutamate release. *Proc Natl Acad Sci U S A* **101**, 9441–9446.

Nonvesicular release of neurotransmitters

Cotrina ML, Lin JH, Alves-Rodrigues A, Liu S, Li J, Azmi-Ghadimi H, Kang J, Naus CC, Nedergaard M (1998) Connexins regulate calcium signaling by controlling ATP release. *Proc Natl Acad Sci U S A* **95**, 15735–15740.

Takano T, Kang J, Jaiswal JK, Simon SM, Lin JH, Yu Y, Li Y, Yang J, Dienel G, Zielke HR, Nedergaard M (2005) Receptor-mediated glutamate release from volume sensitive channels in astrocytes. *Proc Natl Acad Sci U S A* **102**, 16466–16471.

Control of brain microcirculation

Mulligan SJ, MacVicar BA (2004) Calcium transients in astrocyte endfeet cause cerebrovascular constrictions. *Nature* **431**, 195–199.

Takano T, Tian GF, Peng W, Lou N, Libionka W, Han X, Nedergaard M (2006) Astrocyte-mediated control of cerebral blood flow. *Nat Neurosci* **9**, 260–267.

Zonta M, Angulo MC, Gobbo S, Rosengarten B, Hossmann KA, Pozzan T, Carmignoto G (2003) Neuron-to-astrocyte signaling is central to the dynamic control of brain microcirculation. *Nat Neurosci* **6**, 43–50.

Neuronal–glial interactions (Chapter 6)

Tripartite synapse

Araque A, Parpura V, Sanzgiri RP, Haydon PG (1999) Tripartite synapses: glia, the unacknowledged partner. *Trends Neurosci* **22**, 208–215.

Haydon PG (2001) GLIA: listening and talking to the synapse. *Nat Rev Neurosci* **2**, 185–193.

Volterra A, Haydon P, Magistretti P, Eds (2002) *Glia in Synaptic Transmission*. Oxford University Press, Oxford.

Volterra A, Meldolesi J (2005) Astrocytes, from brain glue to communication elements: the revolution continues. *Nat Rev Neurosci* **6**, 626–640.

Volterra A, Steinhauser C (2004) Glial modulation of synaptic transmission in the hippocampus. *Glia*, **47**, 249–257.

Neuronal–glial synapses

Jabs R, Pivneva T, Huttmann K, Wyczynski A, Nolte C, Kettenmann H, Steinhauser C (2005) Synaptic transmission onto hippocampal glial cells with hGFAP promoter activity. *J Cell Sci* **118**, 3791–3803.

Lin SC, Bergles DE (2004) Synaptic signaling between neurons and glia. *Glia* **47**, 290–298.

Functions of astroglia (Chapter 7)

Development and neurogenesis

Alvarez-Buylla A, Garcia-Verdugo JM, Tramontin AD (2001) A unified hypothesis on the lineage of neural stem cells. *Nat Rev Neurosci* **2**, 287–293.

Doetsch F (2003) The glial identity of neural stem cells. *Nat Neurosci* **6**, 1127–1134.

Mori T, Buffo A, Gotz M (2005) The novel roles of glial cells revisited: the contribution of radial glia and astrocytes to neurogenesis. *Curr Top Dev Biol* **69**, 67–99.

Potassium buffering

Kofuji P, Connors NC (2003) Molecular substrates of potassium spatial buffering in glial cells. *Mol Neurobiol* **28**, 195–208.

Kofuji P, Newman EA (2004) Potassium buffering in the central nervous system. *Neuroscience* **129**, 1045–56.

Water homeostasis
Simard M, Nedergaard M (2004) The neurobiology of glia in the context of water and ion homeostasis. *Neuroscience* **129**, 877–96.

Glial regulation of synaptic transmission
Allen NJ, Barres BA (2005) Signaling between glia and neurons: focus on synaptic plasticity. *Curr Opin Neurobiol* **15**, 542–548.
Auld DS, Robitaille R (2003) Glial cells and neurotransmission: an inclusive view of synaptic function. *Neuron* **40**, 389–400.
Pascual O, Casper KB, Kubera C, Zhang J, Revilla-Sanchez R, Sul JY, Takano H, Moss SJ, McCarthy K, Haydon PG (2005) Astrocytic purinergic signaling coordinates synaptic networks. *Science* **310**, 113–116.
Rochon D, Rousse I, Robitaille R (2001) Synapse–glia interactions at the mammalian neuro-muscular junction. *J Neurosci* **21**, 3819–3829.

Functions of oligodendroglia and Schwann cells (Chapter 8)

Baumann N, Pham-Dinh D (2001) Biology of oligodendrocyte and myelin in the mammalian central nervous system. *Physiol Rev* **81**, 871–927.
Corfas G, Velardez MO, Ko C-P, Ratner N, Peles E (2004) Mechanisms and roles of axon–Schwann cell interactions. *J Neurosci* **24**, 9250–9260.
Miller RH (2002) Regulation of oligodendrocyte development in the vertebrate CNS. *Prog Neurobiol* **67**, 451–467.
Sherman DL, Brophy PJ (2005) Mechanisms of axon ensheathment and myelin growth. *Nat Rev Neurosci* **6**, 683–690.

Glial pathology (Chapters 9, 10)

General glial pathology
Seifert G, Schilling K, Steinhauser C (2006) Astrocyte dysfunction in neurological disorders: a molecular perspective. *Nat Rev Neurosci* **7**, 194–206.

Astrogliosis
Pekny M, Nilsson M (2005) Astrocyte activation and reactive gliosis. *Glia* **50**, 427–434.

Wallerian degeneration
Ehlers MD (2004) Deconstructing the axon: Wallerian degeneration and the ubiquitin–proteasome system. *Trends Neurosci* **27**, 3–6.
Koeppen AH (2004) Wallerian degeneration: history and clinical significance. *J Neurol Sci* **220**, 115–117.

Microglia

Kreutzberg GW (1996) Microglia: a sensor for pathological events in the CNS. *Trends Neurosci* **19**, 312–318.

Streit WJ, Ed (2002) *Microglia in the degenerating and regenerating CNS*, Springer-Verlag, New York.

Streit WJ (2002) Microglia as neuroprotective, immunocompetent cells of the CNS. *Glia* **40**, 133–139.

van Rossum D, Hanisch UK (2004) Microglia. *Metab Brain Dis* **19**, 393–411.

Microglial motility

Davalos D, Grutzendler J, Yang G, Kim JV, Zuo Y, Jung S, Littman DR, Dustin ML, Gan WB (2005) ATP mediates rapid microglial response to local brain injury in vivo. *Nat Neurosci* **8**, 752–758.

Nimmerjahn A, Kirchhoff F, Helmchen F (2005) Resting microglial cells are highly dynamic surveillants of brain parenchyma in vivo. *Science* **308**, 1314–1318.

Ischaemia

Nedergaard M, Dirnagl U (2005) Role of glial cells in cerebral ischemia. *Glia* **50**, 281–286.

Lin JH, Weigel H, Cotrina ML, Liu S, Bueno E, Hansen AJ, Hansen TW, Goldman S, Nedergaard M (1998) Gap-junction-mediated propagation and amplification of cell injury. *Nat Neurosci* **1**, 494–500.

Walz W, Klimaszewski A, Paterson IA (1993) Glial swelling in ischemia: a hypothesis. *Dev Neurosci* **15**, 216–225.

Spreading depression

Martins-Ferreira H, Nedergaard M, Nicholson C (2000) Perspectives on spreading depression. *Brain Res Rev* **32**, 215–234.

Walz W, (1997) Role of astrocytes in the spreading depression signal between ischemic core and penumbra. *Neurosci Biobehav Rev* **21**, 135–142.

Alzheimer's disease

Nagele RG, Wegiel J, Venkataraman V, Imaki H, Wang KC (2004) Contribution of glial cells to the development of amyloid plaques in Alzheimer's disease. *Neurobiol Aging* **25**, 663–674.

Streit WJ (2004) Microglia and Alzheimer's disease pathogenesis. *J Neurosci Res* **77**, 1–8.

Wyss-Coray T, Loike JD, Brionne TC, Lu E, Anankov R, Yan F, Silverstein SC, Husemann J (2003) Adult mouse astrocytes degrade amyloid-beta in vitro and in situ. *Nat Med* **9**, 453–457.

Amyotrophic lateral sclerosis

Barbeito LH, Pehar M, Cassina P, Vargas MR, Peluffo H, Viera L, Estevez AG, Beckman JS (2004) A role for astrocytes in motor neuron loss in amyotrophic lateral sclerosis. *Brain Res Rev* **47**, 263–74.

Pain

Tsuda M, Inoue K, Salter MW (2005) Neuropathic pain and spinal microglia: a big problem from molecules in "small" glia. *Trends Neurosci* **28**, 101–107.

Multiple sclerosis

Barnett MH, Sutton I (2006) The pathology of multiple sclerosis: a paradigm shift. *Curr Opin Neurol* **19**, 242–247.

Ludwin SK (2006) The pathogenesis of multiple sclerosis: relating human pathology to experimental studies. *J Neuropathol Exp Neurol* **65**, 305–318.

Ruffini F, Chojnacki A, Weiss S, Antel JP (2006) Immunobiology of oligodendrocytes in multiple sclerosis. *Adv Neurol* **98**, 47–63.

Vanishing white matter disease

van der Knaap MS, Pronk JC, Scheper GC (2006) Vanishing white matter disease. *Lancet Neurol* **5**, 413–423.

HIV

Li W, Galey D, Mattson MP, Nath A (2005) Molecular and cellular mechanisms of neuronal cell death in HIV dementia. *Neurotox Res* **8**, 119–134.

Peruzzi F, Bergonzini V, Aprea S, Reiss K, Sawaya BE, Rappaport J, Amini S, Khalili K (2005) Cross talk between growth factors and viral and cellular factors alters neuronal signaling pathways: Implication for HIV-associated dementia. *Brain Res Rev* **50**, 114–125.

Epilepsy

Fellin T, Haydon PG (2005) Do astrocytes contribute to excitation underlying seizures? *Trends Mol Med* **11**, 530–533.

Kang N, Xu J, Xu Q, Nedergaard M, Kang J (2005) Astrocytic glutamate release-induced transient depolarization and epileptiform discharges in hippocampal CA1 pyramidal neurons. *J Neurophysiol* **94**, 4121–4130.

Tian GF, Azmi H, Takano T, Xu Q, Peng W, Lin J, Oberheim N, Lou N, Wang X, Zielke HR, Kang J, Nedergaard M (2005) An astrocytic basis of epilepsy. *Nat Med* **11**, 973–981.

Schizophrenia, bipolar disorders and other psychiatric disorders

Cotter DR, Pariante CM, Everall IP (2001) Glial cell abnormalities in major psychiatric disorders: the evidence and implications. *Brain Res Bull* **55**, 585–595.

Mitterauer B (2004) Imbalance of glial–neuronal interaction in synapses: a possible mechanism of the pathophysiology of bipolar disorder. *Neuroscientist* **10**, 199–206.

Mitterauer B (2005) Nonfunctional glial proteins in tripartite synapses: a pathophysiological model of schizophrenia. *Neuroscientist* **11**, 192–198.

Gliomas

Chung WJ, Lyons SA, Nelson GM, Hamza H, Gladson CL, Gillespie GY, Sontheimer H (2005) Inhibition of cystine uptake disrupts the growth of primary brain tumors. *J Neurosci* **25**, 7101–7110.

McFerrin MB, Sontheimer H (2006) A role for ion channels in glioma cell invasion. *Neuron Glia Biol* **2**, 39–49.

Ransom CB, O'Neal JT, Sontheimer H (2001) Volume-activated chloride currents contribute to the resting conductance and invasive migration of human glioma cells. *J Neurosci* **21**, 7674–7683.

Sontheimer H (2003) Malignant gliomas: perverting glutamate and ion homeostasis for selective advantage. *Trends Neurosci* **26**, 543–549.

Author Index

Glial Neurobiology: A Textbook   Alexei Verkhratsky and Arthur Butt
© 2007 John Wiley & Sons, Ltd   ISBN 978-0-470-01564-3 (HB); 978-0-470-51740-6 (PB)

Subject Index

Glial Neurobiology: A Textbook   Alexei Verkhratsky and Arthur Butt
© 2007 John Wiley & Sons, Ltd   ISBN 978-0-470-01564-3 (HB); 978-0-470-51740-6 (PB)